John K. Crellin
Fernando Ania

Professionalism and Ethics in Complementary and Alternative Medicine

Pre-publication
REVIEWS,
COMMENTARIES,
EVALUATIONS...

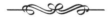
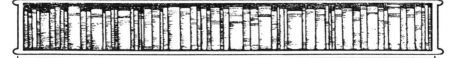

More pre-publication
REVIEWS, COMMENTARIES, EVALUATIONS . . .

"John Crellin and Fernando Ania are educated and well-learned in the formalities of medicine, pharmacy, and history, and now, through this timely study, they are to be placed in the forefront among ethicists. Today alternative/complementary medicine both conflicts and cooperates with traditional medicine. The authors provide scholarly analysis and just plain common sense. Crellin and Ania balance the humors of yellow bile, black bile, and just plain bile in an equilibrium of scholarship that should reach not only students and practitioners of medicine and medical providers, whatever their ilk, but the informed general public as well. Whatever we are, we are or will be patients. How do we deal with open-ended questions, e.g., `Am I getting enough vitamin E or zinc?' `How can homeopathic remedies be unsafe when such minute quantities are employed?' The authors assert that professional obligations transcend legal requirements. Their approach is current and broadly conceived. An easily flowing text is buttressed by references that are up-to-date, most of them since the late 1990s. The current issues in the United Kingdom, Canada, and the United States are addressed. What is a professional health care provider and what are his or her obligations? Diverse views are presented and logical, balanced conclusions are drawn. The concluding section on case histories follows the Hippocratic practice of presenting principles through real-life experiences."

John Riddle, PhD
Head, Department of History;
President, American Institute
for the History of Pharmacy,
North Carolina State University,
Raleigh

The Haworth Integrative Healing Press
An Imprint of The Haworth Press, Inc.
New York • London • Oxford

Professionalism and Ethics in Complementary and Alternative Medicine

THE HAWORTH INTEGRATIVE HEALING PRESS
Ethan Russo
Editor

The Last Sorcerer: Echoes of the Rainforest by Ethan Russo

Professionalism and Ethics in Complementary and Alternative Medicine by John K. Crellin and Fernando Ania

Cannabis and Cannabinoids: Pharmacology, Toxicology, and Therapeutic Potential by Franjo Grotenhermen and Ethan Russo

Modern Psychology and Ancient Wisdom: Psychological Healing Practices from the World's Religious Traditions edited by Sharon G. Mijares

Professionalism and Ethics in Complementary and Alternative Medicine

John K. Crellin
Fernando Ania

The Haworth Integrative Healing Press
An Imprint of The Haworth Press, Inc.
New York • London • Oxford

Published by

The Haworth Integrative Healing Press, an imprint of The Haworth Press, Inc., 10 Alice Street, Binghamton, NY 13904-1580.

The Cunning Man by Robertson Davies. Used by permission, McClelland and Stewart, Ltd. The Canadian Publishers. Used with the permission of Pendragon Ink.

DILBERT © UFS. Reprinted by permission.

Quotation from I. K. Zola in A. A. Alonzo. "Health Behavior: Issues, Contradictions, and Dilemmas." Reprinted from *Social Sciences and Medicine* 37(8):1019-1034. Copyright 1993, with permission from Elsevier Science.

Letters from Alice Nowlan to Theodore Bacmeister, Theodore Bacmeister Papers, Illinois State Historical Library, Springfield, Illinois. Reprinted by permission.

Excerpts from Floyd Skloot's essays "Home Remedies" and "Healing Powers," in *The Night-Side: Chronic Fatigue Syndrome and the Illness Experience*. Reprinted with permission of the author and Story Line Press (<www.storylinepress.com>).

B. M. Berman and J. P. Swyers, "Establishing a Research Agenda for Investigating Alternative Medical Interventions for Chronic Pain," *Primary Care*, 1997, 24:743-758. Reprinted by permission.

Cover design by Anastasia Litwak.

Library of Congress Cataloging-in-Publication Data

Crellin, J. K.
   Professionalism and ethics in complementary and alternative medicine / John K. Crellin, Fernando Ania.
      p. cm.
   Includes bibliographical references and index.
   ISBN 0-7890-1225-1 (alk. paper)—ISBN 0-7890-1226-X (alk. paper)
   1. Alternative medicine specialists—Professional ethics. I. Ania, Fernando. II. Title.

R733 .C743 2002
174'.2—dc21
                                                                2001039102

CONTENTS

Foreword   xi
Raoul Andersen

Preface   xv

Introduction: What to Consider   1

Geographical Coverage and Our Readership   2
Organization of Our Material   4
Being a Professional   5
Health Care Concepts and Beliefs   8
Conventional Medical Attitudes   8
The Future   10
Terminology   10

**PART I: THE CURRENT SCENE—PUBLIC
AND PROFESSIONAL ISSUES**

Chapter 1. Introduction: A Complicated Setting   17

Chapter 2. Scrutinies   19

From the Government   19
From the Medical and Allied Health Professions   20
From Complementary/Alternative Practitioners   28
From the Public   32
General Comments on Future Directions   34

Chapter 3. Changing the Health Care Paradigm?   41

Introduction   41
Values in Health Care   42
Economic Issues   44
Antimedicine/Antiscience, Antigovernment, Anti-Big
    Business   47
Two Cultures, Beliefs About Disease, Holism, and Health   50
Integration   59

Chapter 4. Standards of Care: A Need for Critical Skills   71

Standards of Care, the Courts, and Complementary/
    Alternative Medicine   71

Safety and Standards   73
Critical Evaluation; Historical Pedigrees   80
Quality and Standardization of Preparations   83
Efficacy, Effectiveness, and Placebos   85

Chapter 5. Regulation by Legislation or Self-Regulation?   95

Dietary Supplements and Regulations: Diverse Attitudes   95
Statutory Regulation or Self-Regulation?   97
Education   99
Complementary/Alternative Education for Mainstream
   Practitioners   102
Research   103
Licensing   103
Disciplinary Measures   105

PART II: PROFESSIONALISM

Chapter 6. Professionalism: Many Faces   111

Introduction: Diverse Views   111
Authority and Power   114
Oaths and Codes   122
Modern Bioethics   128

**Chapter 7. Public Expectations of Practitioner Roles
and Responsibilities   145**

As a Communicator   148
As a Scientist   159
As a Healer   160
As a Team Player and Gatekeeper   163
As a Health Advocate   168
Closing Comment   170

**PART III: PROFESSIONAL/ETHICAL ISSUES
IN EVERYDAY PRACTICE—CASE HISTORIES/
READINGS**

Introduction   177

1. Sarah and Her Otitis Media   181

Issues   181
Questions and Comments   182
Some Further Comments   188
Other Conditions   189

2. Mr. O'Grady and DHEA — 191

Issues — 191
Questions and Comments — 192

3. Narratives: Listening to Patients — 195

Issues — 195
Questions and Comments — 202

4. Difficult Professional Relationships — 207

Issues — 207
Questions and Comments — 208

5. Mr. L: The Dilemmas of Multicultural Health — 211

Issues — 211
Questions and Comments — 214

6. The Environment and Connections — 217

Issues — 217
Questions and Comments — 218

7. Testimonials and Advertising by Practitioners — 221

Issues — 221
Questions and Comments — 224

8. Making Diagnoses — 227

Issues — 227
Questions and Comments — 228

9. Prescribing and Selling Remedies — 231

Issues — 231
Questions and Comments — 231

10. Critical Appraisal: Toxicities and Clinical Trials — 235

Issues — 235
General Comments — 237

11. A Chronic Condition: Rheumatism — 239

Issues — 239
Questions and Comments — 241

12. Cancer   **245**

    Issues   245

    Questions and Comments   247

Index   **253**

ABOUT THE AUTHORS

Dr. John K. Crellin holds British qualifications in both medicine and pharmacy. He also holds a PhD in the history and philosophy of science. His principal interest is self-care, particularly the role of complementary medicine. His publications range widely on the history of medicine and pharmacy as well as on herbal medicine and home medicine in general. He has taught undergraduate, graduate, medical, and complementary/alternative medical students in the United Kingdom, the United States, and Canada. His present position is John Clinch Professor of the History of Medicine at Memorial University of Newfoundland; he gives frequent public and professional talks on complementary/alternative medicine. His books include *"By the Patient and not by the Book": Constancy and Change in Small Town Doctoring* (with P. I. Crellin); *Herbal Medicine Past and Present* (with J. Philpott); *Home Medicine: The Newfoundland Experience; Alternative Health Care in Canada: Nineteenth- and Twentieth-Century Perspectives* (co-edited with R. Andersen and J. Connor); and *Healthways—Newfoundland Elders: Their Lifestyles and Values* (with R. R. Andersen and B. O'Dwyer).

Fernando Ania, ND, HD, is Founder and President of the Homeopathic College of Canada and Clinical Director of a busy teaching clinic. He also runs his own private practice in Toronto. He is a graduate of the Ontario College of Naturopathic Medicine and received his HD from the Ontario Homeopathic Association. Dr. Ania began his studies with a focus on Eastern philosophy and continues to explore and research alternative and preventative methods of treatment with a focus on homeopathic medicine. Dr. Ania is Founder, President, and Dean of the International Academy of Homeopathy and former President of the Ontario Homeopathic Association. He has been interviewed and featured in newspapers, magazines, and radio/television programs on alternative and complementary medicine. Dr. Ania is active on the speaking circuit and gives lectures and seminars to medical associations, hospitals, business groups, universities, and colleges around the world. His research paper "The Effect of Constitutional Hydrotherapy on White Blood Cell Count" was published in 1988.

Foreword

This book is a cutting-edge examination of professionalism and ethics issues in the relationship between mainstream and what is often termed "alternative" medicine. Its authors, John K. Crellin and Fernando Ania, bring expert knowledge from decades of intensive study of these issues. From the perspective of a social anthropologist interested in the social-cultural side of health, illness, and health care, the authors illustrate complexities and dynamics inherent in our rapidly shrinking world. The history of health, illness, and care reflects societal and cultural origins such as the rise of industrial capitalism and globalization. Once "exotic" knowledge and practices of other cultures, and their somehow arcane Western culture counterparts, now figure increasingly in renewed talk of "traditional knowledge" and mind, body, and self in health and healing. One result is a dynamic health care culture rife with competing ideas, practices, and uncertainties.

During the past two centuries the growth of the scientific approach to medicine, its popularization, and rising health care expectations helped channel the pluralistic health and illness belief systems and practitioners of the past into two major streams, one to center stage, the other to the margins. In Western nations, the former, often termed "conventional" or "bioscientific" medicine, emerged to become near empyrean in organization, legitimacy, exclusiveness, and power. The other—commonly known lately under such umbrella terms as traditional, alternative, and complementary medicine (e.g., traditional Chinese medicine such as acupuncture), and its practitioners, have been diverse, less exclusive, less organized, often maligned, and struggle for respectability.

In third world societies, of course, that which is considered alternative medicine in the West is commonly the primary health care recourse, and biomedicine, if at all accessible, is the exception. In the West, despite its social and cultural diversity and often, marginality, alternative medicine has the characteristics and attraction of a health care social or even countercultural movement. This movement is widely promoted in popular media that champion more natural, self-directed, and/or spiritual lifestyles, products, and healing practices. Both the healthy and the ill resort to them, either alone or in combination with reliance upon mainstream medicine. This dual dependency often occurs without the knowledge or cooperation of practitioners on both sides. The consequence for patients is a heightened uncertainty, if not risk to their health. Increasingly, of course, many mainstream practitioners have added various alternative methods (such as acupuncture, acupressure, homeopathy, chiropractic, and dietary health supplements) to their practices. What does this say of practitioners and their professionalism?

Similar to other social and cultural constructions created in history's ebb and flow, boundaries between different health care belief systems and ideas inspire uncertainty and debate involving cultural values. Issues of rationality, invasiveness, accessibility, utility, efficacy, and especially professional responsibility and ethics figure in this book. These, as with all cultural things, are subject to change. Ideas and practices based upon scientific evidence or biomedicine are neither always convincing nor enduring. In recent decades the once-seeming juggernaut of mainstream medicine is often questioned and constrained by public institutions. Notwithstanding excitement over such medical innovations as human genomic investigation and its promises, it is no longer heresy to question its limits and excesses. The shifting ground of societal requirements and public values that have created respect for ethnic cultural diversity, accessibility, and patient autonomy command new health care thinking. A different professional knowledge is expected, one that is more aware of patient expectations and practices, and that recognizes the pros and cons of alternative healing approaches as well as what constitutes ethical conduct. The idea of professionalism in health care occupations is no exception, as what follows demonstrates.

Professionalism and Ethics in Complementary and Alternative Medicine is directed at students and practitioners of both complementary/alternative and conventional health fields. It thrusts both groups of health care practitioners into situations in which they must respond to ethical issues that coexist in the health care field today. If they are to live up to their claims for legitimate professional status, both must realize the need to develop a different consciousness, one that responds to ethical dilemmas created by their own ideas and practices.

Exploring this vast and varied field, practitioners of both health care streams are faced with numerous ethical issues that must be addressed. Doing so against a historical background discussion, we are led to existing evidence in both scientific and other literature, including rapidly changing Web site sources, accessible to both patients and practitioners. Readers will relish the illumination of issues in the many concrete cases and contexts presented. Placed in the position of practitioners and the dilemmas they face, readers will recognize issues otherwise ignored.

Finally, this book contributes to the discourse on trends in health care now running parallel, and their complex relationships to our society and institutions. The authors help us understand unrecognized and debated problems, disagreements, and concessions compromising these relationships, as in complementary practices that many practitioners and patients may now take for granted. The authors' discussion is practical and systematic, and their analytic approach provides a sound framework for judgment of local issues. It is a challenging guide to intelligent judgment and resolution of many ethical issues in the health care field today.

Raoul Andersen, PhD
Professor of Anthropology
Memorial University of Newfoundland

Preface

This volume grew out of a short course on ethics and law at the Homeopathic College of Canada in Toronto. The students, some embarking on second careers, raised countless questions and concerns that often reflected their diverse backgrounds. For example, "Am I investing in a profession that will flourish?" "How deep are the tensions between conventional and alternative medicine?" "Are the values and ethics I have been taught in nursing school the same as those of homeopathy?" "How serious is the competition I face from those who have learned homeopathy by correspondence?"

Students of medicine, nursing, and other conventional health professions also have many questions. In medical schools, such interest is fed by growing numbers of courses on complementary and alternative medicine. These have come at a time when many physicians are changing attitudes toward what, at one time, was widely seen as quackery.

With all the questions and changes, plus the fact that professional/ethical issues have been getting more formal attention in health care education (perhaps mostly in medicine), we felt the need for a broadly based volume to bring together a wide range of issues that center on professionalism. We hope that the present result—prepared by educators from a school of medicine and from a homeopathic college—will not only serve as a textbook for students and practitioners of complementary and alternative medicine but also for a variety of other readers: mainstream health care professionals, patients, and the public in general. Aside from specific issues for practitioners, all readers will gain a better understanding of the complexity of issues that face the future of health care, the concerns of complementary and alternative medicine, and efforts to integrate it with mainstream medicine.

In preparing this book we wish to thank students over many years, especially Karolyn Bradbury, who have asked pointed questions about trends and developments in health care; colleagues who have encouraged and challenged us, particularly Raoul Andersen, an anthropologist at Memorial University of Newfoundland; various practitioners who have offered us insights into their practices, including physician Wael Shublaq, an immigrant to North America, who shared his dilemmas while successfully taking up an acupuncture practice as he was waiting to get a medical license; the eagle eye of JDC; and Rosalind Nichols, who would not have survived without a word processor as she cheerfully dealt with change after change as the manuscript developed. Special thanks go to Peg Marr, Amy Rentner, Dawn Krisko, and Mary Beth Madden of The Haworth Press for their diligence and care in the preparation of the manuscript.

Introduction: What to Consider

The past twenty years or so of burgeoning interest in complementary/alternative health care has spawned vigorous debates and ethical concerns. One authoritative view is that "complementary therapies require an even greater appreciation of ethical concerns [than conventional medicine], given the nonmeasurable, nonrational dimensions of holistic practice." This is particularly the case "in therapies which do not have a highly technical skill base, where ethical, rather than therapeutic, complaints are likely to give greater cause for concern."[1]Our discussions focus not only on specific ethical matters of conduct and moral judgments, but also more generally on the nature and responsibilities of professionalism at a time when many complementary/alternative organizations are striving for professional recognition. Although being a professional in health care means different things to different people, a central consideration is how to provide the highest level of quality care. While this is perhaps an obvious truism, we emphasize that it means more than just diagnosis and treatment. It also embraces humane judgment supported by an infrastructure of practitioners who maintain standards of education and practice; who take responsibility to improve the status quo in health care; and who identify, analyze, and resolve professional/ethical problems in everyday clinical practice.[2]

Professional/ethical issues are not new in complementary/alternative medicine. After all, "alternative" approaches to health care have a long, tortuous history covering countless practices. These include the Royal Touch (healing by the touch of a king, common up to the end of the eighteenth century); nineteenth-century "botanic" medicine; Dr. John Harvey Kellogg and his work, from 1876, at the celebrated Battle Creek Sanitarium (recently used loosely in the novel and film *The Road to Wellville,* which satirizes "cults" of hygiene, nutrition, and cleanliness); and "toe-twisting" by the twentieth-century Canadian physician Mahlon Locke.[3] However, until recently, ethical matters that attracted public interest were likely to be the disciplining of physicians who practiced alternative medicine, or an episode in the medical profession's many efforts to curb "quackery." Nowadays, in sharp contrast, a wide range of issues with professional/ethical implications is being publicly scrutinized. They include

1. the safety, quality, and efficacy of many complementary/alternative treatments and procedures;
2. the making of diagnoses by unregulated practitioners;
3. the existence of quackery, misleading labeling and hype (e.g., such headlines as "Ginkgo biloba miracle cure");
4. the presence of factionalism and divisiveness among complementary/alternative practitioners often reflecting their uneven education and qualifications; and
5. the questionable standards of many regular physicians in their practice of complementary and alternative medicine.

A central purpose of this book is to make clear that numerous concerns about health care—nowadays being explored more systematically than ever before in mainstream medical and nursing education—are essential considerations for *all* practitioners providing health care. After all, as others have said, "alternative medicine and conventional medicine share some important goals," central to which is the development of ethical care and effective therapeutic relationships.[4] Calls from medical educators, who believe that "professionalism must be taught" to, for example, medical students merely reinforce the importance of these matters.[5] We are also concerned with the issue of integration of mainstream and complementary/alternative medicine; although we explicitly discuss integration in places, much else of what we say indicates that, if it is to happen in a constructive and meaningful way, countless issues have to be addressed. Unquestionably, a key issue is a need for all health care practitioners to understand the positions and attitudes of the "other side," to which we hope this volume will contribute. This introduction indicates the organization of our material and key themes.

GEOGRAPHICAL COVERAGE AND OUR READERSHIP

"Complementary medicine is booming worldwide," proclaimed a 1996 medical article that usefully surveyed a number of countries.[6] Unquestionably, one of the most fascinating aspects of the complementary/alternative scene is that it is a social movement in all Western countries. It is because of common features that we draw on material from both sides of the Atlantic, and occasionally from elsewhere, such as Australia.[7] Of course, there are also national differences, but cross-cultural comparisons are always instructive. For instance, they prompt reflection on overly familiar situations at home and raise questions about, for example, how far the emphasis on individual autonomy—which characterizes so much of bioethics in the United States—is acceptable on the global stage.[8] Comparisons also reveal that a specific event can make a significant impact on the direction of complementary/alternative medicine in one region or country; examples include the establishment of the U.S. Office of Alternative Medicine in 1991 (now called the National Center for Complementary and Alternative Medicine) and the British government's decision (1992) to allow general practitioners to make payments out of their National Health Service Practice budgets for the referral of patients to complementary practitioners.[9]

Similarly, broad sociocultural comparisons raise various considerations. One U.S. contributor to 1998 Canadian discussions on regulating natural health products offered his view that while the cultures of the United States and Canada are very similar, a big difference was the latter's consultative process between government and users. "This did not happen in the States. The FDA [Food and Drug Administration]," he said, threw "industry down the stairs time and time again, refusing to talk about these issues, dictating, telling industry 'this is the way it's going to be. You can't sell this.' End of conversation."[10] Although numerous Canadians may have no higher opinion of Canadian authorities than many Americans have of the FDA, arguably a more accommodating attitude to complementary/alternative medicine may well exist in Canada than in the United States. Overall, a neutral or central position is more common "north of the Border," a sense of compromise seemingly part of Canadian culture.[11]

This book is intended for a wide readership:

1. Complementary/alternative practitioners and students who practice (or will practice) with or without a license
2. Licensed medical practitioners, nurses, pharmacists, and others in conventional health fields, as well as respective students

3. Social science students, patients, and the general public who want a better understanding of the responsibilities of those who offer complementary/alternative care.

Groups (2) and (3) include those who are skeptical of complementary/alternative medicine, but everyone in health care needs to understand its significance and impact on health care in general.

ORGANIZATION OF OUR MATERIAL

The first part of this volume outlines current issues and trends. Part II builds on this by looking more specifically at professionalism and relevant ethical matters. Both parts set the stage for further reflection in Part III, through case histories and readings, on various matters that emerge in everyday complementary and alternative practice. In organizing the volume, we considered commencing with specific discussions on professionalism and ethics (Part II). After all, books on ethics commonly begin with "foundations" or ethical theories. However, we believe that the ability to identify and analyze professional/ethical (including legal) issues—or potential ones—and to implement decisions, demands a broad understanding of relevant everyday health care issues and trends. An ability to see the "big picture" and to identify where value judgments are needed are important considerations in professionalism and in evaluating many ethical dilemmas. We must also emphasize that those practicing complementary/alternative medicine need to be aware of problems beyond their own specialty. Hence, Part I pulls together numerous issues characterizing the current scene: differing attitudes toward government, science, and big business; reforms in health care; patients' beliefs; concepts such as reductionism and holism; consumerism; conflicting opinions about the need for regulation, the safety of herbal products, the qualifications of physicians who practice alternative medicine; and much more. Unfortunately, few of these matters are dealt with formally in either mainstream or complementary/alternative medicine. Although we cannot pursue any topic exhaustively, we set the stage for both personal reflection and classroom discussion. We document in some detail our sources from the rapidly growing literature for further reading.

It is noteworthy that the big picture of complementary/alternative care does not reveal a well-ordered canvas, but a rather disordered patchwork of diverse issues that seemingly reflects what is called our postmodern era, a view that characterizes much of present-day society in terms of multiplicity, fragmentation, and uncertainty.[12] At the same time this prompts calls for bioethicists to pay more attention to the complexity of social and cultural influences that shape ethical situations and their interpretation.[13] Moreover, such attention may help with understanding how "an ordinary problem becomes a bioethical problem."[14] An appreciation of the big picture also helps with a *systematic* evaluation of a professional/ethical dilemma. Our approach covers evaluating, where relevant,

1. data or facts (scientific, clinical, legal, and sociocultural);
2. a patient's beliefs and concepts about health and disease and how these may differ from mainstream views;
3. a practitioner's personal values, attitudes (including ethics), and biases that may affect decision making;
4. ethical theories and codes of ethics that guide one's thinking; and
5. how best to negotiate sensitively ethical decisions with patients and families.

Obviously everyone involved in decision making has particular responsibilities to consider systematic approaches. For instance, apparent ethical problems may evaporate in the face of a full knowledge of facts (e.g., that a practice is safe, not dangerous), while an understanding of a patient's concepts of health and disease can facilitate communication and negotiation. Of course, this does not mean that a simple right or wrong answer will be found to a dilemma, but a careful analysis can suggest why one answer may be preferred over another, as well as allowing practitioners to justify to themselves and others a difficult decision among the countless uncertainties of medical practice.

BEING A PROFESSIONAL

A central question behind much discussion in this volume is, What exactly does it mean to be a professional? As we will see, this is not particularly easy to answer, partly because perceptions of what a profession does, and how it tries to define itself, change over time. Moreover, even practitioners respond in different ways to the question. However, as is elaborated in Part II, professionalism today must at least recognize and respond to what the public expects of its practitioners. This includes not only paying attention to such long-standing values as compassion and honesty, but also to certain roles such as being a "person," a "communicator," a "scientist," a "healer," a "team player," a "gatekeeper," and a "clinician." Complementary/alternative practitioners may say that much of this reflects public expectations of regular physicians alone and does not apply to them. However, the roles must be given very serious consideration by *all* health care practitioners in today's societies when following a cardinal principle—serving the *best interests* of patients by providing quality care. Of course, just what is meant by a patient's best interests begs such questions as, "Who determines what is best?" and "What criteria are used?"

That answers to such questions, as all ethical questions, rarely find a consensus of views serves as a reminder of the particular responsibilities of all practitioners (conventional and complementary/alternative). Here we just refer to the need to understand professional and personal values and their relevance to being a "good" practitioner. Professional values include the responsibility to acquire *knowledge, skills,* and appropriate *attitudes.* In fact, appropriate attitudes—a prerequisite for diligently acquiring and applying knowledge and skills—have become an increasingly conspicuous public concern as when physicians fail to show sensitivity toward patients.[15] Fears also exist that professional attitudes and responsibilities are being overly shaped by legal rather than ethical considerations. The following two events raise questions for all practitioners about professional attitudes.

First, a 1998 British newspaper article, titled "Doctors 'close ranks' over negligence cases," dealt with the plight of British parents without the legal right to receive full details about an accidental hospital death of their child. The article stated that, following a court decision that maintained the status quo (the Will Powell judgment), the General Medical Council told doctors that they "have a moral obligation, *if not a legal one,* to be frank with parents."[16]

Second, the disciplining of a physician, prior to his 1998 election as President of the Canadian Medical Association, received widespread attention largely because of initial efforts to conceal the physician's identity. In addition, the physician—after his identity was revealed—attracted scrutiny when he argued that limits exist to professional disciplining of physicians, a view that questioned the heart of professional self-regulation.[17] We believe, as do others, that professional/ethical practice is not bound by the law and commonly must rise above it.

One of our core arguments is that appropriate professional attitudes for ethical practice can be fostered by self-reflection—by understanding one's biases, weaknesses, and strengths. As practitioners and students look at themselves, it may well be to see where they stand with regard to two ends of a spectrum of worldviews; at one end is a group who are predisposed to rely only on objective facts, and at the other end are those who are equally sensitive to subjectivity and to an appreciation that medicine is as much an art as a science.[18]

As a way to develop self-reflection, we suggest that practitioners may usefully consider a tradition—one fostered by the humanities—of employing a mirror, so to speak, as a tutorial device to look at oneself, to pursue self-knowledge, to "know thyself."[19] Some observers suggest, perhaps unkindly, that physicians in particular are not prone to examine their professional selves, and, if they do so, it is somewhat narcissistically. Yet practitioners' understanding of themselves may well influence the way they practice. Quality of care can be enhanced, especially in such nontechnology aspects as counseling patients, offering patient education, giving adequate information for informed consent, and defusing tensions patients may feel over regular and complementary/alternative treatments.

The theme of reflections extends to considering the images and perceptions of practitioners held by patients and the public in general. Are physicians viewed too negatively? Are holistic alternative practitioners either overly glamorized or dismissed altogether? Above all, writers and artists explore, as do health care practitioners, the human condition, albeit in a different way. We notice writers, from Robertson Davies to Floyd Skloot, who offer insights and values from the humanities; after all there are strong arguments for saying that the humanities can contribute much to quality care and humane judgment; some even say that "medicine is really something like applied humanities."[20] In places, we notice, too, historical context not so much to offer the interpretations of historians, but to provide a sense of constancy and change that helps to place current issues in perspective. Unfortunately, within the space of a single volume, we cannot pursue the humanities' perspectives on professionalism as much as we would wish, but we suggest further reading in many endnotes.

HEALTH CARE CONCEPTS AND BELIEFS

A further reason for looking at current issues is to consider the various meanings attached to such terms as holism, health, and reductionism in medicine, as well as the significance of ideologies (e g , antiscience) found today. Different meanings given to terms and concepts often lead to misunderstandings and ethical dilemmas. This is part of the two worldviews or two cultures we have noted. One culture represents those who wish to change health care to "a better and more natural way" and the other comprises those who believe that effective health care must continue to be based on "science." In fact, different ideologies and concepts—often accentuated by the very different languages and discourses of medicine, spirituality, and metaphysics—can divide sharply the supporters of complementary/alternative medicine and those who view it as quackery or, at best, nothing more than "placebo medicine." Although it is difficult for most people to stand outside their own culture, we hope that our discussions will foster efforts to understand other points of view. This includes a consideration of whether a trend exists, noticeable by 2000, toward a growing middle ground between the two cultures.

CONVENTIONAL MEDICAL ATTITUDES

Of all the issues we touch on about professions, concerns about them being self-serving constantly appear. Indeed, a commonplace interpretation by sociologists of professional groups is that they are able to regulate their market conditions by creating a monopoly both through controlling entry to the group and controlling the specialized knowledge that is to be used.[21] Of particular relevance to our discussions is whether the attacks on complementary/alternative medicine from conventional medical organizations stem from efforts to stifle competition, rather than from careful analysis of its contribution to health care.

Conflicts between serving the profession rather than the public have been examined in recent years by many sociologists, as summarized in M. Saks' *Professions and the Public Interest: Medical Power, Altruism and Alternative Medicine.*[22] Saks indicates that the actions of a profession often fail to match its professed concern with the public interest. He explores fully nineteenth- and twentieth-century opposition to acupuncture from British doctors and concludes that their response was colored by professional self-interest, backed by a professional ideology.

Another example, one that raises questions about the sincerity of medicine's expressions about public safety, is the British Medical Association's vigorous nineteenth- and twentieth-century campaign against the "quack medicine trade," while its own journal, the *British Medical Journal,* accepted advertisements—needed for the journal's financial future—for the offending products.[23] And, more recently, a 1997 U.S. court found that the American Medical Association, the American College of Radiology, and the American College of Surgeons joined together, conspiratorially, from the mid-1960s through the mid-1980s, to induce "their members to forego any form of professional, research, or educational association with chiropractors."[24]

Nowadays, physicians' attitudes toward complementary medicine are less resolute and more varied. However, we wonder whether a medical backlash is growing (certainly noticeable by the late 1990s if not before), at least among professional medical organizations. There is no shortage of disparaging comments in the medical press as complementary/alternative medicine becomes more popular. A 1998 editorial in *The New England Journal of Medicine* stated:

> what most sets alternative medicine apart, in our view, is that it has not been scientifically tested and its advocates largely deny the need for such testing. . . . Now, with the increasing interest in alternative medicine, we see a reversion to irrational approaches to medical practice, even while scientific medicine is making some of its most dramatic advances.[25] (M. Angell and J. P. Kassirer, "Alternative Medicine—The Risks of Untested and Unregulated Remedies," *New England Journal of Medicine,* 1998, 339: 839-841. Copyright 1998 Massachusetts Medical Society. All rights reserved.)

The *Canadian Medical Association Journal* went further in saying, "No amount of evidence will convince the flat-earthists [referring to supporters of complementary/alternative medicine] that the world is round."[26] In many ways, such sentiments go beyond long-standing attacks on quackery, and, arguably, reflect physicians' concerns about their loss of medical power in all Western countries. For instance, new Dutch legislation, which came into force in 1998 and ended "the monopoly of the Dutch medical profession," resonates with legislation in North America.[27] Clearly this has implications for the structure of health care in the future.

THE FUTURE

Not only does knowledge of the contemporary scene help to identify professional/ethical issues, but it also helps with making informed responses to the question, "Where are we going?"

Although few commentators anticipate the eclipse of complementary/alternative medicine in the near future, a 1998 article by a professor of complementary medicine, Edzard Ernst, "The Rise and Fall of Complementary Medicine," reflected the hopes of many that its "popularity had reached its peak."[28] However, the view was readily challenged.[29] Certainly in 2000, there are no signs of fading interest in complementary/alternative medicine, and the many reasons for its popularity suggest it is firmly established. Indeed, various factors indicate that, as a social movement with considerable momentum, it is unlikely to fade in the near future.[30] On the other hand, many variables and crosscurrents make forecasting the future difficult, especially the level of integration that may or may not take place. For instance, what will be the outcome of two currently conflicting trends, one toward greater standardization and accountability in all aspects of health care, and the other, supported by legislation, toward greater acceptance of patients' autonomy and choices?

TERMINOLOGY

We close this introduction with comments on terms. First, our use of "complementary/alternative" medicine. Emerging from extensive discussions (published and otherwise) in recent years, the term "alternative medicine" has become less favored than "complementary and alternative medicine," or, particularly in the United Kingdom, just "complementary." Complementary and alternative indicates that therapies are used either as adjuncts to (i.e., to complement) conventional medicine, or, deliberately, albeit to a lesser extent, as "alternatives."[31] However, the same therapy may be used both ways, hence our use of the slash in complementary/alternative.

Second, "mainstream" or "conventional" medicine is referred to in countless ways when contrasted with complementary/alternative, for instance, regular, conventional, official, traditional, Western medicine, allopathy, biomedicine, and scientific medicine. We consider that these terms generally carry overtones of bias; for instance, biomedicine and scientific medicine can imply absence of any humanistic orientation. In the text we generally use mainstream or conventional as being relatively impartial.

Third, a comment on our use of "patients" rather than "clients" or "consumers." Which term should be used in health care today leads to vigorous debate. Although "clients" acknowledges a person's autonomy, we have chosen what some describe as the obsolete term, "patients"; this is largely because it reminds us that imbalance in authority and power between practitioners and those who seek their help remains common—the "white coat" phenomenon is well established and persists—despite the current emphasis on patient empowerment and consumerism. Imbalance of power must be constantly recognized and given due ethical attention.

A further problem in preparing a text on contemporary complementary/alternative medicine is that it is a fluid scene with a very large number of modalities, often grouped as indigenous, nutrition-based, herbal, manual, mind/body, biochemical, and miscellaneous. Moreover, some are being seen in places as becoming mainstream (e.g., acupuncture and chiropractic), whereas others may well be viewed as fringe (e.g., iridology) even within some complementary/alternative circles. Prayer, too, or more generally spirituality, is often viewed as complementary/alternative, whereas for many people it has long been an integral part of their life and health. However, amid this diverse scene, and with specific issues associated more with certain practices (e.g., matters of safety), there are countless professional/ethical matters common to all modalities.

Some specific issues emerge from the diversity of practitioners, especially when some are physicians and others nonphysicians. The latter are often referred to as "lay" or "professional" (as is common in homeopathy). The latter terms are hardly satisfactory, however, since "lay" practitioners may well have far more training and experience in their modality than any physician; moreover, "professional" can suggest that physicians are not professional when practicing a complementary/alternative modality. When we must make a distinction we generally use, for example, MD (or medically qualified)-homeopath or MD-acupuncturist, which at least recognizes dual qualifications.

NOTES

1. J. Stone and J. Matthews, *Complementary Medicine and the Law*, Oxford: Oxford University Press, 1996, p. 204.

2. For specifying the relationship between quality of patient care and ethics: P. Singer, "Recent Advances: Medical Ethics," *British Medical Journal*, 2000; 321, 282-285. (This journal, since 1988, has been titled *BMJ*, which we use henceforth.)

3. In large measure, the history of alternative medicine is written as a history of quackery or as the history of sectarian medicine. Its battles with conventional medicine are rightly emphasized, but, unfortunately, little attention is given to assessing its contributions to health care. Representative titles that prompt questions rather than an overall negative tone include R. Porter, *Health for Sale: Quackery in England, 1660-1850,* Manchester: Manchester University Press, 1989. For Canada, in a different vein, J. K. Crellin, R. R. Andersen, J. T. H. Connor, *Alternative Health Care in Canada: Nineteenth- and Twentieth-Century Perspectives,* Toronto: Canadian Scholars Press, 1997.

While T. C. Boyle, *The Road to Wellville,* New York: Viking Penguin, 1994, is a good example of the efforts to highlight the gullible and to steer them away from nutty approaches to health care, it is also a useful tool to prompt discussion on attitudes.

4. J. Sugarman and L. Burk, "Physicians' Ethical Obligations Regarding Alternative Medicine," *Journal of the American Medical Association,* 1998; 280, 1623-1625. (This journal, since 1960, has been titled *JAMA,* which we use henceforth.)

5. For example, S. R. Cruess and R. L. Cruess, "Professionalism Must Be Taught," *BMJ,* 1997; 315, 1674-1677.

6. *BMJ,* 1996; 313, 131-134. For a useful review of European countries, see European Commission, *Cost Action B4: Unconventional Medicine,* Luxembourg: Office for Official Publications of the European Communities, 1999.

7. P. A. Komesaroff, "Use of Complementary Medicines: Scientific and Ethical Issues," *Medical Journal Australia,* 1998; 169, 180-181.

8. For example, R. Baker, "Negotiating International Bioethics: A Response to Tom Beauchamp and Ruth Macklin," *Kennedy Institute of Ethics Journal,* 1998; 8, 423-453.

9. See R. W. Davey, "A Perspective on Complementary Medicine," *Medico-Legal Journal,* 1997; 65(2), 65-85.

10. House of Commons Standing Committee on Health Minutes, March 24, 1998, p. 44. We quote from this 1997-1998 Canadian House of Commons Committee review of natural health products in various places in this volume. This is because it offers verbatim documentation of diverse views widespread in the late 1990s, not only in Canada, but also throughout North America and beyond. Page numbers are to House of Commons Web site version: <http://www.parl.gc.ca/l.../CommitteeEvidence.asp?Language=E&Parliament=1&Joint=O&CommitteeID=1> (accessed September 2001 for access to meetings November 6, 1997 to June 4, 1998).

11. Differences between the United States and Canada explored in J. K. Crellin, R. R. Andersen, and J. T. H. Connor, *Alternative Health Care in Canada* (3), 257-261.

12. For discussion on the concept of modernity and whether complementary/alternative medicine is part of it: M. Saks, "Medicine and Complementary Medicine: Challenge and Change," in G. Scambler and P. Higgs, eds., *Modernity, Medicine and Health: Medical Society Toward 2000,* New York: Routledge, 1998, pp. 198-215.

13. This is the thrust of much discussion in R. DeVries and J. Suhadi, eds., *Bioethics and Society: Constructing the Ethical Enterprise,* Upper Saddle River, NJ: Prentice-Hall, 1998.

14. R. DeVries and P. Conrad, "Why Bioethics Needs Sociology," in DeVries and Suhadi, eds., *Bioethics and Society: Constructing the Ethical Enterprise,* Upper Saddle River, NJ: Prentice-Hall, 1998, pp. 233-257.

15. As an example, the concerns have become conspicuous in the United Kingdom. The General Medical Council has taken a lead in responding to public concerns, see *General Medical Council Annual Review,* 1998.

16. *Guardian Weekly,* December 13, 1998, p. 11 (italics added).

17. *National Post,* November 14, 1998, p. A8; *The Medical Post,* 1998; 34 (October 6), 1, 49. "Reddoch reflects on CMA post," *The Medical Post,* 1999; 35 (May 18), 1, 66. The disciplining was upheld.

18. For some discussion, H. Wulff, "The Two Cultures of Medicine: Objective Facts versus Subjectivity and Values," *Journal of the Royal Society of Medicine,* 1999; 92, 549-552.

19. This theme is pursued in a stimulating book, Jonathan Miller, *On Reflection,* London: National Gallery Publications, 1998. See J. K. Crellin, "On Reflection," *MUNMED* [Faculty of Medicine, Memorial University of Newfoundland], 1999, 11, 3.

20. For example, C. Shooner, "The Ethics of Learning from Patients," *Canadian Medical Association Journal,* 1997; 156, 535-538. Comments made by a general physician, albeit commonplace in medical humanities literature. Compare also, E. P. Scarlett, "What Is a Profession?" in R. Reynolds and J. Stone, eds., *On Doctoring,* New York: Simon and Schuster, 1991, pp. 113-119, who sees literature as an aspect of the Seven Pillars of Wisdom of professionalism.

21. For overview in relation to health care: M. Saks, "Professionalism and Health Care," in D. Field and S. Taylor, eds., *Sociological Perspectives on Health, Illness and Health Care,* Oxford: Blackwell Science, 1998, pp. 174-191.

22. M. Saks, *Professions and the Public Interest: Medical Power, Altruism and Alternative Medicine,* London: Routledge, 1995.

23. See P. Bartrip, "Secret Remedies, Medical Ethics, and the Finances of the British Medical Journal" in R. Baker, ed., *The Codification of Medical Morality: Historical and Philosophical Studies of the Formalization of Western Medical Morality in the Eighteenth and Nineteenth Centuries,* Dordrecht: Kluwer Academic Publishers, 1995, Volume 2, 191-204.

24. See N. Gevitz. "The Chiropractors and the AMA: Reflections on the History of the Consultation Clause," *Perspectives in Biology and Medicine,* 1989; 32, 281-

299. For the saga of chiropractic, the medical profession, and the state in Ontario, see "Negotiating a Scope of Practice for Chiropractic: An Overview of the Ontario Case," in York University Centre for Health Studies, *Complementary and Alternative Practices and Therapies,* Toronto: York University Centre for Health Studies, 1999, pp. 151-199.

25. M. Angell and J. P. Kassirer, "Alternative Medicine—The Risks of Untested and Unregulated Remedies," *New England Journal of Medicine,* 1998; 339, 839-841.

26. I. F. Tannock and D. G. Warr, "Unconventional Therapies for Cancer: A Refuge from the Rules of Evidence?" *Canadian Medical Association Journal,* 1998; 159, 801-802.

27. See R. M. J. Schepers and H. E. G. M. Hermans, "The Medical Profession and Alternative Medicine in the Netherlands: Its History and Recent Developments," *Social Science and Medicine,* 1999; 48, 343-351. For North America, one of the most significant acts is the Regulated Health Professions Act of Ontario (see Licensing, in Chapter 5).

28. E. Ernst, "The Rise and Fall of Complementary Medicine," *Journal of the Royal Society of Medicine,* 1998; 91, 235-236.

29. For comments on the British scene, see R. Tonkin, "The 'Boom' in Complementary Medicine," *Journal of the Royal Society of Medicine,* 1998; 91, 399.

30. For a recent background discussion emphasizing disquiet with science and medicine, see R. Lewinsohn, "Medical Theories, Science, and the Practice of Medicine," *Social Science and Medicine,* 1998; 46, 1261-1270. Confidence that complementary and alternative medicine will not fade is expressed in R. C. Kessler, R. B. Davis, D. F. Foster, M. I. Van Rompay, E. E. Walters, S. A. Wilkey, T. J. Kaptuchuk, D. M. Eisenberg, "Long-Term Trends in the Use of Complementary and Alternative Medical Therapies in the United States," *Annals of Internal Medicine,* 2001: 135, 262-268.

31. A recent U.S. study indicated only a small number of users compared with those who used it in a complementary manner: B. G. Druss and R. A. Rosenheck, "Association Between Use of Unconventional Therapies and Conventional Medical Services," *JAMA,* 1999; 282, 651-656.

PART I:
THE CURRENT SCENE—
PUBLIC AND PROFESSIONAL ISSUES

Chapter 1

Introduction: A Complicated Setting

How did nineteenth-century alternative practitioners deal with being labeled unorthodox or quacks? Did they see themselves as health reformers? Did they wish for more social standing? Are the same issues current today? The dichotomy between mainstream medicine and other forms of medical care has deep roots that anchor attitudes today.

Historians, like sociologists, generally see physicians' concerns with maintaining monopoly as key reasons for this dichotomy.[1] It was particularly significant that, as mainstream medicine came to rely more on observing pathology and on science during the nineteenth century, it had new reasons for attacking "nonscientific" practices, which it commonly labeled as quackery. Fears of quackery continue to be fostered today, either specifically or as part of the general opposition to complementary/alternative medicine. One respected U.S. commentator wrote (1997), "as scientific medicine advanced and regulatory law gained greater power, pseudoscience also grew so that in our own day larger sums are expended on quackery than ever before in our nation's experience."[2] The "dangers" are constantly highlighted by, for instance, media reports and the well-known, U.S.-based Quackwatch Internet site.[3] Thus a long-standing specter continues to overshadow complementary/alternative care and prompts warnings to "beware" of it. This feeds worries about, for instance, the safety of various products, erratic licensing/nonlicensing of complementary/alternative practitioners in many jurisdictions, as well as countless ethical issues. If the latter are rarely as emotive as abortion and euthanasia, they are common, everyday issues affecting quality of care. Moreover, as ethicists often say, it is important to prevent small matters (e.g., misunderstandings in communication)—often due to the colossal amount of conflicting advice that exists—becoming major "fire-alarm" situations.

Historical perspective helps us, too, not only to understand reasons for the present rather chaotic state of complementary/alternative medicine in many Western countries, but also why current interest is probably not a "flash in the pan." Many observers see a strong parallel between the enthusiasm for alternative therapies in the nineteenth century with the current widespread usage. They see a temporary fading of interest during the first half or so of the twentieth century as due primarily to public and government enthusiasm for new scientific developments in medicine, which aided the medical profession to develop virtual control in health care. It is no surprise that the rapid growth of complementary/alternative care in recent years—partly due to concerns with mainstream medicines—is being scrutinized by the medical profession. In fact, much of the scrutiny (also by governments, allied health professions, the general public, and practitioners of complementary/alternative medicine) is, as we now consider, constructive. It is certainly important for all practitioners in health care to appreciate the many concerns and questions, trends and counter trends, social and political issues, reflected in today's evaluations. Such matters are at the heart of how a profession "negotiates" the politics of health care.

NOTES

1. The history of complementary/alternative medicine is substantial. A few relevant texts to issues raised in this volume: S. E. Cayleff, *Wash and Be Healed: The Water-Cure Movement and Women's Health,* Philadelphia: Temple University Press, 1987; R. Cooter, ed., *Studies in the History of Alternative Medicine,* New York: St. Martin's Press, 1988; H. L. Coulter, *Divided Legacy: A History of the Schism in Medical Thought,* Berkeley: North Atlantic, 1994, 4 volumes.; J. K. Crellin, R. R. Andersen, and J. T. H. Connor, eds., *Alternative Health Care in Canada: Nineteenth- and Twentieth-Century Perspectives,* Toronto: Canadian Scholars' Press, 1997; R. C. Fuller, *Alternative Medicine and American Religious Life,* New York: Oxford University Press, 1989; M. Saks, *Professions and the Public Interest: Medical Power, Altruism and Alternative Medicine,* London: Routledge, 1994; W. I. Wardwell, *Chiropractic: History and Evolution of a New Profession,* St. Louis: Moseby, 1992.

2. J. H. Young, "Health Fraud: A Hardy Perennial," *Journal Policy History,* 1997; 9, 117-140.

3. Web site address of Quackwatch: <http://www.quackwatch.com> (accessed September 2001).

Chapter 2

Scrutinies

FROM THE GOVERNMENT

Just what should be a government's role in health care, of which complementary/alternative medicine is but one aspect, has long raised heated debate. Indeed, in modern times, due to such episodes as the dramatic congenital side effects associated with expectant mothers taking thalidomide in the early 1960s, arguments that governments have a responsibility to protect the health of the public have strengthened. Nowadays, in "protecting the public and promoting health," governments face the dilemma that they must also respect the autonomy of individuals. Some commentators paint the scene as public interest versus patient autonomy. Trying to find the "right" balance vexes not only legislators, but also stakeholders in complementary/alternative care. The latter are commonly concerned over government biases, and many believe that the medical profession's special influence on government bureaucracies—once very evident—still exists. Some hold, too, a long-standing view of political economists that the state primarily serves the needs of business, rather than of the individual (including in health matters). When worries have erupted over the safety of particular herbs (e.g., chaparral, comfrey, or ephedra) differences of opinion between governments, scientists, and users often center on charges that bureaucracies pay too much attention to vested interests.

Given all the issues, and especially public lobbying for less control of dietary supplements (also commonly known as nutraceuticals), it is not surprising that governments have, in recent years, actively looked for new policies.[1] It is noteworthy that in the United States, prior to the Dietary Supplement Health and Education Act of 1994 (and in the wake of the 1991 establishment of the government-funded Office of Alternative Medicine) "congress received more mail on the [Act] than on any subject since the Vietnam War."[2] In Canada, following the "hot" issue of herbal remedies during the 1997 election, a

Canadian House of Commons Standing Committee on Health investigated, with much public consultation, the place of natural health
products in Canadian society.[3] The committee's recommendation to
establish a new regulatory framework for such products was accepted
by the Canadian government.[4] In one sense, as noted in Chapter 5,
under Dietary Supplements and Regulations, the U.S. and Canadian
governments have been led to compromise legislation.

Government scrutiny, in the early 2000s, extends to licensure, or at
least setting frameworks for licensing. This varies from jurisdiction
to jurisdiction (see Chapter 5, Research). Here we merely note that
the complementary/alternative practitioner must recognize that the
inconsistent practices of various jurisdictions is problematic. This is
particularly so in the United States and Canada, where licensing is a
state or provincial, not federal, matter. Clearly, questions of professional responsibility arise for all practitioners as they contribute to
debate on how governments can best balance public safety with the
autonomy, the freedom of choice, of individuals.

FROM THE MEDICAL AND ALLIED
HEALTH PROFESSIONS

Long-standing and ongoing vigorous opposition to complemen-
tary/alternative medicine from the medical profession has already
been emphasized. Many see this as resulting less from critical scrutiny than from the ideology of rejecting "nonscientific" practice. As
said, the strengthening of medical opposition to alternative medicine
in the nineteenth century was linked to the profession's commitment
to new medical science, and to an increasingly science-based education that fostered a reformist zeal. This, in forging a new "improved"
medicine, contributed to new ethical precepts that prohibited physicians from consulting with alternative practitioners.[5]

Although it is wrong to assume that the medical profession has ever
had a totally uniform voice, a very conspicuous level of diverse opinion
presently exists over whether complementary/alternative medicine
should be excluded from or incorporated (perhaps after reformula-
tion) into conventional medicine. Although criticism from physicians
about complementary/alternative medicine—commonly on the basis
that it is "unscientific" in approach, at best a placebo action or merely
for the "worried well"—remains very noticeable, many physicians

added one or more complementary/alternative modalities to their regular practice between the 1980s and early 2000s. These physicians on both sides of the Atlantic—usually general practitioners (but also some specialists)—are persuaded by empirical evidence that patients are helped; they often ignore the "unscientific" theory (acupuncture and homeopathy are commonly mentioned), and suggest that Western science will ultimately explain the practice.[6] Further, their approach, albeit often reshaping practices (e.g., so-called "modern acupuncture" is a Westernized approach based on conventional anatomy and physiology), may well fit the holistic philosophy associated with much complementary/alternative medicine (compare Box 2.1).

Other physicians, although not practicing complementary/alternative care themselves, at least believe that it should be available for

---

BOX 2.1. "But Many of My Professional Colleagues Swore at Me"

Already a legend was growing up about me. It was suggested that I used unconventional methods and there is nothing a professional group mistrusts so nervously as it does anything that appears unconventional, and that has not been thoroughly written up in the journals. It may be quackery. Worse still, it may be effective. And if it is both quackery and effective it is utterly hateful.

The reasons why many physicians have added complementary/alternative practices to mainstream medicine are diverse. Famed novelist Robertson Davies captures many issues in his highly recommended novel, *The Cunning Man* (1994). In this "autobiography" of a physician, Robertson Davies offers many insightful thoughts about the interface—often a challenging one—between conventional and complementary medicine. Although a regularly licensed physician, the novel's central character, Dr. Jonathan Hullah, became known for a distinctive practice in which he attached much importance to the psychosocial aspects of care. As Hullah said:

Many of my patients, in their phrase, swore by me. But many of my professional colleagues swore at me, for I appeared to them to be a heretic about health. . . . My dictionary says that a quack is somebody who professes a knowledge of which he is ignorant; but I profess nothing of the sort—I simply profess a knowledge of which a great many of my professional colleagues are ignorant. I suppose I might call it humanism.*

*The dilemmas of shifting into unconventional practice appear in many places in R. Davies, *The Cunning Man*, Toronto: McClelland and Stewart, 1994, but especially pp. 245-249. Used with the permission of Pendragon Ink.

their patients. A British study (1998) on access to complementary/ alternative medicine in general practice stated that recent studies of general practitioners, hospital doctors and medical students have "shown a softening of attitudes and a general integration of complementary therapy within traditional practice."[7] This supported earlier studies (e.g., 1994) that claimed three-quarters of U.K. doctors thought that some form of complementary medicine should be provided by the National Health Service.[8] This is only slightly higher than a U.S. study (also 1994) indicating that more than 60 percent of community physicians referred patients to complementary/alternative practitioners.[9] Studies in 1998 of U.S. physicians found that many psychobehavioral and lifestyle therapies appear to have become accepted as part of mainstream medicine, that chiropractic and acupuncture were apparently gaining acceptance, despite low levels of training, and that substantial personal use occurred.[10] A further 1998 "review of the incorporation of complementary and alternative medicine by mainstream physicians" in various countries found that acupuncture had the highest rate of physician referral (43 percent) followed by chiropractic (40 percent) and massage (21 percent).[11]

An important aspect of physician involvement is the influential local, national, and international physician-promoters of complementary/alternative medicine; examples from the 1990s range from Dr. Andrew Weil, a U.S. media star, commonly introduced by his "Harvard-trained" pedigree, to Dr. Jozef Krop of Toronto, a practitioner of environmental medicine, whose protracted disciplinary hearings with the Ontario College of Physicians and Surgeons became a public cause célèbre.[12]

It is also clear that many physicians, often in positions of influence, believe that alternative/complementary medicine should no longer be ignored, even by skeptics. Surveys of usage of complementary/alternative therapies have now appeared in many specialty medical journals, for instance, "arthritis" (see case history/reading 11), rhinosinusitis,[13] Parkinson's disease,[14] and women's cancer (see case history/reading 12). Studies also exist on patients with acute disease as well as on various chronic conditions which are well known to encourage usage.[15] Moreover, there is also the incorporation, albeit slow and uneven, of complementary/alternative concepts and practices into hospital practice. In many ways, this responds to today's maxim of "patient-centered care," which, it has been said, leaves hospitals with no choice but to offer complementary treatments: "If you believe in the primacy of patients making their own decision and you believe in the fundamental of informed consent, you cannot deny them access to this treatment."[16] However, struggles commonly exist over such matters as whether unlicensed practitioners can practice in hospitals.

The diversity of views about the complementary/alternative medicine movement underscores questions for all practitioners about responsibilities to patients, to oneself and to their profession. Physicians need to be able to justify on experiential, experimental, or theoretical grounds, the positions they take toward nonmainstream practices: (1) pro, (2) con, (3) sitting on the fence, or (4) fear of the "slippery slope" (for instance, that the dominance of scientific medicine will be lost).

In terms of a physician's responsibilities to the medical profession, it must be said that physicians who have embraced a complementary/alternative modality into their practice have often been intemperate in remarks about colleagues who have "not seen the light." In other contexts, the same physicians may reveal an aloofness, if not arrogance—perhaps fed by a sense of medical power—to nonmedically qualified complementary/alternative practitioners. Despite growing acceptance by many colleagues, MD-homeopaths, for example, are still marginalized by the medical profession in general. Indeed, an apparent late-1990s medical backlash emerged (at least among medical organizations) to the "inexorable tide" of complementary/alternative care. Aside from specific attacks from leading medical journals already noted, and media attacks from time to time, new by-laws and regulations have been established for the physician-practice of complementary/alternative medicine by various physician licensing boards in North America.[17] Although such new regulations are a distinct change from the long-standing professional ethic that physicians must not consult with "irregulars," the regulations seem to be galvanized, at least in part, by a significant curbing by new "external" legislation (state and provincial) of medicine's self-regulatory powers. The thrust of this—with patients' rights at the center—is to prevent medical boards from disciplining physicians for practicing a complementary/alternative modality so long as certain conditions are met.[18] In the United States, federal legislation is perhaps moving in the same direction, though an Access to Medical Treatment Act has still to be passed.[19]

We now offer some details of regulatory responses from selected licensing boards, to raise questions in the reader's mind about medical attitudes and to highlight further the nature of professional/ ethical tensions facing many licensed physicians who wish to add complementary/alternative medicine to their armamentarium. A constant consideration is whether "official" professional values are always in the best interests of patients. The new regulations also prompt the question: To what extent should the new regulations for physicians serve as models for non-medically qualified practitioners endeavoring to professionalize their specialty?

In contrast to some recently published ethical statements (e.g., the general advice from the American College of Physicians; see Box 2.2), some of the most detailed and exacting directions (called by some "cavalier paternalism") come from Alberta's licensing authority, the College of Physicians and Surgeons of Alberta.[20] In 1997, the College reacted to the Alberta Medical Profession Amendment Act (in force on October 1, 1996), which stated:

> A registered practitioner shall not be found guilty of unbecoming conduct or be found to be incapable or unfit to practice medicine or osteopathy solely on the basis that the registered practitioner employs a therapy that is non-traditional or departs from prevailing medical practices, unless it can be demonstrated that the therapy has a safety risk for the patient unreasonably greater than the prevailing treatment.[21]

In new regulations, the College mandated a detailed schedule that every Alberta physician must follow in order to practice complementary care. Key points are as follows. First, a "registered medical practitioner shall not provide complementary health care therapy(s) to some or all of his or her patients until approval from the Registrar after a physician submits his or her intention to provide specific treatments."

To support an application, a physician must provide suitable documentation of his or her abilities, ranging from postgraduate education, certification, continuing education, and "the standards of practice of the complementary therapy accepted by educational centers where the therapy is taught." If such documentation is unavailable,

---

BOX 2.2. Ethics for Physicians

The following statement from the American College of Physicians "Ethics Manual,"* can be compared with the more complex directives of the Canadian medical licensing boards considered in the text.

Alternative Treatments

Alternative or complementary medicine is a common term for health practices that generally are not available from U.S. physicians, are not offered in U.S. hospitals, and are not widely taught in U.S. medical schools. The physician should not abandon the patient who elects to try an alternative treatment. Requests by patients for alternative treatment require balancing the medical standard of care with a patient's right to choose care on the basis of his or her values and preferences. Such a request warrants careful attention from the physician. Before advising a patient, the physician should ascertain the reason for the request: for example, whether it stems from dissatisfaction with current care. The physician should be sure that the patient understands his or her condition, standard medical treatment options, and expected outcomes.

The physician should encourage the patient requesting alternative treatment to seek literature and information from reliable sources. The patient should be clearly informed if the option under consideration is likely to delay access to effective treatment or is known to be harmful. The physician need not participate in the monitoring or delivery of alternative care to the patient. However, physicians should recognize that some patients may select alternative forms of treatment: this decision alone should not be cause to sever the patient-physician relationship.

---

*American College of Physicians "Ethics Manual," *Annals of Internal Medicine,* 1998; 128, 576-594 (p. 577).

---

the College requires alternative information including "a representative sample of clinical outcomes satisfactory to the Registrar including a comparison with orthodox methods of treatment."

One requirement—considered particularly onerous by many—is that a physician has to sign an agreement to follow the specified practice guidelines. These have also to be followed under "exceptional circumstances":

> The Registrar may permit a registered practitioner who does not hold [general] approval to administer complementary health care therapy(s) to provide the same to a patient who suffers from an imminently fatal, incurable disease as long as the practice

guideline attached hereto is accepted and followed by the registered practitioner.

We cannot detail the information to be recorded as demanded by the practice guidelines—from stating the diagnosis to indicating "the likely effect of the recommended therapy(s) on the patient's functioning in the family and the social and workplace environments." However, we do notice a clause that has aroused particular frustration, namely a mandated "reflection period." Patients must wait seventy-two hours prior to initiation of a complementary/alternative treatment, but if they are not prepared to wait, they must provide the physician with a written request for the immediate initiation of treatment.

The stringent regulations of Alberta can be usefully compared with other jurisdictions in Canada and the U.S. The licensing body of Manitoba issued in 1997 a "formal position of the College with which members shall comply."[22] It covers not only the practice of complementary/alternative medicine by physicians, but also responses physicians may give to questions from patients. With mixed messages, it reminds physicians about the need to recognize the "well-being of patients," that medicine is "rooted in the scientific method," that "ethical physicians are expected to respect the right of informed patients to make decisions with respect to the health services they wish to access," and that the physician has a responsibility to recommend to patients "only those modes of therapy which are consistent with the scientific method." If a physician disapproves of an alternative therapy, or it is potentially harmful, he or she is to counsel the patient accordingly, and not remain silent or nonjudgmental. Moreover, physicians should investigate the available literature to validate unproven remedies through "scientific inquiry." At least (as in Alberta) exceptional circumstances are noted when the gravity of the prognosis and the patient's apparent need for the therapy offset concerns about the harm. Thus the physician has discretion to take into account the patient's need for psychological support.

Somewhat less exacting, if not more liberal policies exist for, for example, Ontario[23] and Texas. The Texas State Board of Medical Examiners 1998 Standards for Physicians Practicing Integrative and Complementary Medicine recognize "that physicians should be allowed a reasonable and responsible degree of latitude in the kinds of therapies they offer their patients [and] that patients have a right to seek integrative or complementary therapies."[24] The guidelines state that a "licensed physician shall not be found guilty of unprofessional conduct or be found to have committed professional failure to practice medicine in an acceptable manner solely on the basis of employing a health care method of integrative or complementary medicine." Exceptions would be if the practice has a safety risk that is "unreasonably greater than the conventional treatment for the patient's medical condition." The guidelines also indicate the points of detail that must be included in a full case record such as "whether conventional medical treatment options have been discussed with the patient and referral input, if necessary."

Even with the sense of more liberal attitudes by the Ontario and Texas Licensing Authorities, all the guidelines reveal tensions. In reflecting a grudging acceptance that complementary/alternative medicine must be acknowledged, the licensing authorities highlight (and some may say contribute to: (1) tensions between being *consistent with the scientific method*—to use the Manitoba phrase—and ethically respecting the decision of a patient who chooses practices that are not consistent with contemporary science; and (2) tensions between serving the best interests of the patient and maintaining the prevailing professional standards of clinical medicine and their allegiance to science.

Readers will respond differently to the directives of various medical licensing authorities. Some will undoubtedly be frustrated by apparent contradictions; for instance, when some authorities allow physicians to practice chelation therapy even while vigorous criticisms of the practice exist.[25] Others feel that certain directives (especially Alberta's) devalue both an individual physician's professional responsibility and a patient's autonomy. However, the directives do challenge MD-practitioners of complementary/alternative medicine to evaluate and perhaps raise their sometimes minimal educational standards in, say acupuncture or homeopathy. Further, the directives challenge all complementary/alternative practitioners to examine standards and to prompt reflection on their own attitudes towards them.

Nursing and Pharmacy

Space only allows a brief note on two other mainstream professions, nursing and pharmacy, that have increasingly interfaced with complementary/alternative care. Many nurses (and midwives) have been in the forefront as promoters of a wide range of complementary/alternative modalities, but especially therapeutic touch and massage. Although, so far as we know, no nursing licensing authority has established guidelines such as the medical ones considered, some nursing authorities continue to license a nurse who has shifted into full-time practice in certain areas of complementary/alternative care so long as guidelines are fulfilled.[26] At issue, however, is that the standards for doing this are not necessarily clear to the public—e.g., is the nurse equipped to diagnose without special training?—and thus the door is open to potential ethical problems. In fact, concerns have been expressed about the failure of the nursing profession to scrutinize.critically complementary/alternative care.

The same concern would seem to apply to pharmacy, which since the late 1990s has become increasingly involved in the sale of herbs and dietary supplements. Although some jurisdictions are offering guidance to pharmacists, it is hard to see (in 2000) whether these have any general impact on quality care. A clear ethical issue has emerged over conflicts of interest between securing profits and maintaining professional integrity.[27]

FROM COMPLEMENTARY/ALTERNATIVE PRACTITIONERS

If mainstream health professionals express diverse responses to the recent rapid expansion of the complementary/alternative medicine movement, so do its nonmedically qualified practitioners. Polarized views and factionalism are common as reflected in the plethora of complementary/alternative medicine organizations and educational standards. Although discord can be a sign of growth—in fact, some see it as a step toward professionalization—it raises concerns inside and outside the movement. Those striving for professionalism, at least licensing and uniform standards of practice, often find themselves at loggerheads with those who want no regulation. To the often noted resistance to professionalization, we add one small, yet typical instance of two homeopathic groups, both based in Toronto: they gave conflicting opinions to the Canadian House of Commons Standing Committee on Health about the need for provincial licensure for homeopathic practitioners.[28]

Of course some of the discord arises from ingrained views. Did nineteenth-century practitioners see themselves as "health reformers" concerned with changing the overall nature of medical care? Many certainly were as they called for "reform" in therapy (e.g., substituting milder treatments—some "drugless" like water-cure—for "strong" mainstream treatments such as heroic levels of bloodletting). Calls for change also demanded greater emphasis on prevention through, for example, bathing, fresh air, dress reform and much more.[29] Today many complementary/alternative practitioners are concerned with bringing about overall change. This does not yet amount to a conspicuous movement, as most current reform effort by individual practitioners is localized through endeavors to put their internal "house in order" and to bring about harmony through developing regional and national "professional" organizations that speak with one voice.[30]

One trend, however, which may signal broad changes, emerged in the 1990s among at least a conspicuous core of practitioners of complementary/alternative medicine. In homeopathy, for instance, many (especially MD-homeopaths) developed a commitment to finding scientific explanations, just as they ignored the basic classical tenet of vitalism (a doctrine that the functions of a living organism are due to a vital principle or force distinct from physico-chemical reactions).[31] There was a change, too, in attitudes toward the contentious issue of the medical "gold standard," namely the randomized double-blind clinical trial to assess efficacy of treatment. Although physicians have, since the 1960s, seen this approach as central to medicine, complementary/alternative practitioners have commonly felt that the methodologies of such trials (e.g., randomization, double blinding, and the use of placebos) are unsuitable to assess the hallmark of complementary/alternative practices, namely holistic treatment tailored to an individual patient.[32] Talk persists of scientific imperialism on the part of regular medicine; however growing complementary/alternative acceptance by 2000 of conventional scientific standards is linked to the achievement of greater acceptance by the medical establishment and by legislators, as well as to retention of the public standing that complementary/alternative medicine has already attained. Further, some hope it will pave the way for integration with conventional medicine.

Some practitioners are saying that there cannot be variable standards in health care, and that it should no longer be acceptable to rely solely on such subjective statements as "I know it works on my patients." Such views echo those of the U.S. National Center for Complementary and Alternative Medicine, which makes clear that complementary and alternative medicine needs to be investigated using as rigorous, and, in some cases, even more rigorous research methods than the current standard in conventional medicine.[33]

This emphasis on the need for research extends beyond major influential institutions such as the U.S. National Center, to smaller centers such as the U.K. Department of Complementary Medicine at the University of Exeter; its conferences and other activities stress the need for scientific validation.[34] Noteworthy, too, is a new genre of books—often collections of papers written by MDs and PhDs (only some of whom practice complementary/alternative care)—that focus, as titles commonly suggest, on critical appraisal and on accountability in medical research and patient care. Examples are *Complementary/Alternative Medicine: An Evidence-Based Approach* (Mosby, 1999), edited by J. W. Spencer and J. J. Jacobs; *Homeopathy: A Critical Appraisal* (Butterworth-Heinemann, 1998), edited by E. Ernst and E. Hahn; *Science-Based Complementary Medicine* (Royal College of Physicians of London, 1998); and *Complementary Medicine: An Objective Appraisal* (Butterworth-Heinemann, 1996), edited by E. Ernst.

Whether or not this push to validation reflects more the interests of physicians who practice complementary/alternative therapy, or of scientists led by the "carrot" of increasingly available funding to pursue such research, it is evident that new professional responsibilities are emerging for complementary/alternative practitioners to scrutinize their treatment standards.[35] This includes considering the relevance or otherwise of a new (1990s) standard in conventional medicine—albeit one prompting reservations among some physicians— namely "evidence-based" medicine, considered to be a reform or new era in health care as a whole.

Central to evidence-based medicine are critical evaluations of therapeutic interventions based on graded "levels" of evidence. At the top are meta-analyses of relevant gold-standard clinical trials, or a "systematic" review of trials (the latter is undertaken, in a prescribed way, when existing trials are not sufficiently similar in methodology for a meta-analysis). The next level is a single randomized controlled trial, followed by the least acceptable level of evidence, namely, single case histories and anecdotal or word-of-mouth experiences. This critical approach to evidence has already extended to complementary/alternative medicine, and is supported through the international

Cochrane Collaboration with funding from the U.S. National Center for Complementary and Alternative Medicine.[36] The relatively few meta-analyses or systematic reviews of complementary/alternative studies available by the early 2000s raise not only questions about the quality of existing complementary/alternative medicine clinical trials, but also general questions about adequate research methodologies. Thus on acupuncture for asthma, a Cochrane review of seven studies states: "There is not enough evidence to make recommendations about the value of acupuncture in asthma treatment. Further research needs to consider the complexities and different types of acupuncture."[37]

Obviously, increasing professional demands are placed on all practitioners as new assessments of efficacy become accepted. As with many conventional physicians, complementary/alternative practitioners will question carefully the concept of evidence-based medicine, at least of meta-analyses. Physicians have asked: Is there an incongruity between "best available evidence" which is derived from group studies and its application to the care of individuals who may not conform to a group in all respects?[38] To what extent is a "personal significance" factor—namely the different rates of progression of an illness due to a variety of factors—relevant to evaluating clinical research findings for everyday practice.[39]

From all we have said, a clear push exists toward shifting the philosophy of complementary/alternative medicine toward a science-based orientation. The implications of this, as noted in our discussion on integration (see Chapter 3), are far-reaching, perhaps even a "takeover" by MD-complementary/alternative practitioners. This worries many non-MD counterparts who remember that it was, for example, the failure of MD-homeopaths in the U.S. and Canada to maintain homeopathic philosophy and practice standards in the early decades of the twentieth century that, along with the growing public acceptance of medical science, contributed to the virtual demise of homeopathy in North America.

This brings to mind another matter that prompts disagreement, namely complementary/alternative practitioner attitudes to mainstream medicine. In contrast to the growing sensitivity to scientific research implied in our above remarks, "most writing and debate about conventional medicine in the complementary practitioner community is decidedly negative in tone."[40] Divisiveness in health care—which rarely serves a patient's best interests—is currently fostered from both "sides," and complementary/alternative practitioners have as much responsibility as anyone to scrutinize consequences of "bad-mouthing" others, especially in relation to patient care.

FROM THE PUBLIC

We have mentioned that intense lobbying for freedom of choice preceded new U.S. and Canadian policies on nutritional supplements. This, along with the data from various surveys, reflects the existence of a grassroots or populist complementary/alternative medicine movement.[41] The movement is fed, in part, by new resources of medical information, especially the Internet, which as it continues to offer new challenges to traditional medical authority and expertise, will undoubtedly exert more and more influence on health care.[42]

The new sources of information illustrate diverse and inconsistent attitudes toward health. Although overlap and even some apparent contradictions exist among the main reasons listed below for the use of complementary/alternative medicine, it must be remembered that each person has his or her own needs and that these may change during the course of even one illness.[43]

1. Belief in the efficacy of "natural" treatments, and perhaps miracles, if not for cure, then for easing symptoms
2. Experience that a particular modality has been helpful
3. Belief that complementary/alternative medicines and practices "don't hurt you and may help a bit"
4. The attractiveness of many complementary/alternative concepts because they are congruent with popular belief systems, for example, the need for balance in life, for spirituality, or to fulfill ethnic needs—in other words, congruent with personal values
5. The disquiet with various aspects of mainstream medicine, ranging from the inadequacies of treatment for terminal and for chronic conditions ("doctor's medicines are not working") to side effects of treatment and physicians' seemingly insensitive attitudes to patients
6. The desire for more personal control in health and illness, whether it be for minor chronic problems or life-threatening

situations; a belief that one has personal responsibilities in health and illness, making choices and monitoring one's own health (This may become particularly evident as a result of distress, perhaps depression, at the state of one's own health.)

7. The need to reduce health care costs (depending on insurance coverage or lack of it)

8. Belief that, in maintaining health, it is prudent to try out new health ideas, even if it is recognized that scientists disagree about effectiveness (Many people concerned with their health are curious about new ways and have the insurance to pay for their curiosity.)

9. The importance patients attach to the length of office time alternative practitioners generally give to patients, as well as to their emphasis on health promotion

10. The influence of testimonials from relatives, friends, health food store personnel, and the Internet

Linking many of these reasons is a search for "something," for a treatment that can be described as holistic (see the discussion of holism in Chapter 3). Of special interest is the search for spirituality (compare point 4 above). Indeed, the need to fill spiritual emptiness is often considered to be a significant factor behind the interest in complementary/alternative medicine. Certainly few expect to find it in conventional medicine; perhaps this is changing, at least praying for the sick attracts growing interest.[44] Aside from the established place of, for example, faith healing and Christian Science, various complementary/alternative medicine modalities have affinities with New Age interest in the spirituality of Eastern and aboriginal religions that are allied with beliefs in balance and cosmic connections. This, however—especially the New Age sense of pantheism—worries many, and vigorous opposition to complementary/alternative care can often be heard from fundamentalist Christians.

In one sense, our remarks may suggest the grassroots interest in complementary/alternative medicine is largely one of searching for something new, rather than of critical appraisal of what it has to offer. However, it would be wrong to think that there is no critical scrutiny among users. Indeed, by the early 2000s growing concerns over safety and the need for standards (including licensing) were becoming more evident, as were dilemmas in choosing the most appropriate modality for a particular ailment, dilemmas that lead to patients "shopping around."[45]

GENERAL COMMENTS ON FUTURE DIRECTIONS

Our comments so far indicate diverse views on complementary/alternative medicine. Although a distinct polarization exists—explored further when we consider "two cultures"—if we read the signs correctly, the twenty-first century begins with some blurring between the two extremes and growing acceptance of complementary/alternative medicine. Despite some belief that the interest is a fashion that will fade (the "bubble will burst"), it is unlikely that this will happen in the near future, except possibly for certain modalities. It is noteworthy that a 1999 report on "Unconventional Medicine" from the European Commission stated, in the context of legislative trends, that "generally speaking [a trend exists toward the] official recognition that complementary medicines can play an important role within health care systems."[46]

At the same time, trends on both sides of the Atlantic indicate that a significant segment of complementary/alternative medicine users have become more demanding, that they want professional help in making appropriate choices, and that new standards of safety and quality are likely to be implemented in most countries. All practitioners must evaluate their response to such trends, which may well reshape the present scene. They must consider the public expectations of them as professionals, as consumers become more critical of excessive hype, expensive treatments and the confusing diversity of practitioners. The question for many is whether complementary/alternative medicine, despite its handicap of speaking with many voices, will "reform" the climate of health care, especially by effecting greater attention to patient choice, responsibility, equity, and calls for change.[47]

NOTES

1. Unfortunately, the term nutraceutical is defined in various ways, E. Bull, L. Rapport, B. Lockwood, "What Is a Nutraceutical?" *Pharmaceutical Journal,* 2000; 265, 57-58.

2. P. Brevoort, "The U.S. Botanical Market," *HerbalGram,* 1996; (36), 49-57.

3. Statement made by Ms. Aileen Carrol (and others), House of Commons Standing Committee on Health Minutes, November 20, 1997, p. 9.

4. The House of Commons Committee's final report, "Natural Health Products: A New Vision" (November 1998), was in line with an earlier Canadian report, "Draft Regulatory Framework for Natural Health Products: Interim Report of the Advisory Panel on Natural Health Products," February 3, 1998. This came from a panel to advise the Therapeutic Products Programme of Health Canada about the regulatory framework for herbal remedies, including product and establishment licensing, cost recovery, international harmonization, etc.

For government response: "Minister Rock accepts all fifty-three recommendations made in the Standing Committee report on natural health products," <http://www.hc-sc.gc.ca/hpb/onhp/rock_e.html> (accessed September 2001).

5. At least this was formalized in the United States. See R. Baker, ed., "Introduction" in *The Codification of Medical Morality: Historical and Philosophical Studies of the Formalization of Western Medical Morality in the Eighteenth and Nineteenth Centuries*, Dordrecht: Kluwer Academic Publications, 1996, Volume 2, pp. 1-21.

6. For growing non-general practitioner interest, D. Reilly and S. Bawden, "Hospital Consultants' Views on Homeopathy," *Journal Royal Society of Medicine*, 1999; 92, 215; for one physician's attitudes about keeping an open mind about theory, A. J. Rockel, "Scientific Fundamentalism Rides Again," *The Medical Post*, 1999; 35(November 23), 13.

7. A. M. Wearn and S. M. Greenfield, "Access to Complementary Medicine in General Practice: Survey in one UK Health Authority," *Journal of the Royal Society of Medicine*, 1998; 91, 465-470.

8. See M. R. Perkin, R. M. Pearcy, and J. S. Fraser, "A Comparison of the Attitudes Shown by General Practitioners, Hospital Doctors and Medical Students Towards Alternative Medicine," *Journal Royal Society of Medicine*, 1994; 87, 523-525.

9. J. Borkan, J. O. Neher, O. Anson, and B. Smoker, "Referrals for Alternative Therapies," *Journal of Family Practice*, 1994; 39, 545-550. Reports also exist that, elsewhere, alternative medicine is becoming more accepted by the medical profession, e.g., "Alternative Medicine Making Headway with Aussie Docs," *The Medical Post*, 1998; 34 (January 6), 16.

10. B. M. Berman, B. B. Singh, S. M. Hartnoll, B. K. Singh, and D. Reilly, "Primary Care Physicians and Complementary-Alternative Medicine: Training, Attitudes and Practice Patterns," *Journal of the American Board of Family Practice*, 1998; 11, 272-281; M. A. Burg, S. G. Kosch, A. H. Neims, and E. P. Stoller, "Personal Use of Alternative Medicine Therapies by Health Sciences Center Faculty," *JAMA*, 1998; 280, 1563.

11. J. A. Astin, A. Marie, K. R. Pelletier, E. Hansen, and W. L. Haskell, "A Review of the Incorporation of Complementary and Alternative Medicine by Mainstream Physicians," *Archives of Internal Medicine*, 1998; 158, 2303-2310. Compare, also, N. P. Gordon, D. S. Sobel, and E. Z. Tarazona, "Use of and Interest in Alternative Therapies Among Adult Primary Care Clinicians and Adult Mem-

bers in a Large Health Maintenance Organization," *Western Journal of Medicine,* 1998; 153-161, 169.

12. In 1999, after many years, the Disciplinary Committee of the College of Physicians and Surgeons of Ontario found Dr. Krop guilty of professional misconduct for failing to maintain the standard of practice in the management, treatment and care of six patients. (Treatment charts of six patients, 1985-1992, were reviewed.) The Committee emphasized that "'Environmental Medicine' was not the issue being deliberated." Aside from public figures like Weil, various physicians have published testimony to positive roles for complementary/alternative medicine, for example, S. J. Winawer with N. Taylor, *Healing Lessons,* Boston: Little, Brown, 1998. (An oncologist changes attitudes during his wife's cancer.)

13. J. H. Krause and H. J. Krause, "Patient Use of Traditional and Complementary Therapies in Treating Rhinosinusitis Before Consulting an Otolaryngologist," *Laryngoscope,* 1999; 109, 1223-1227.

14. For example, B. V. Manyam and J. R. Sánchez-Ramos, "Traditional and Complementary Therapies in Parkinson's Disease," in G. M. Stern, ed., *Parkinson's Disease: Advances in Neurology,* 1990; 80, 565-574.

15. For example, J. Armishaw and C. C. Grant, "Use of Complementary Treatment by Those Hospitalized with Acute Illness," *Archives Diseases Childhood,* 1999; 81, 133-137.

16. Comments about Toronto's Sunnybrook Health Sciences Centre: A. Elash, "Move into Hospital Sector Another Sign of Complementary Medicine's Growing Popularity," *Canadian Medical Association Journal,* 1997; 157, 1589-1592.

17. Although evidence for a backlash comes from certain organizations of professional medicine, elements exist within the "ranks," e.g., B. Sibbald, "New Group Sets Sights on Herbal Medicine," *Canadian Medical Association Journal,* 1999; 161, 583. The medical backlash, of course, adds to the long-standing high level of concern and language of "battles," e.g., C. Ramos-Remus and A. S. Russell, "Alternative Therapies—Medicine, Magic or Quackery. Who Is Winning the Battle?" *Journal of Rheumatology,* 1997; 24, 2276-2279.

18. M. H. Cohen, *Complementary and Alternative Medicine Legal Boundaries and Regulatory Perspectives,* Baltimore: Johns Hopkins Press, 1998, pp. 92-95. Patients' rights are often raised in the complementary/alternative medicine literature. As one example, "Know Your Patients' Rights," *Hope,* 1997; 1(1), 4.

19. "Access to Medical Treatment Act H.R. 2635" (through <http://www.holistic alternatives.net/hr_2635.htm> (accessed September 2001). The medical opposition to the Act poses the question, Should Americans have access to a medical treatment if there are individuals who can personally testify that it is valuable?

20. For quote, "cavalier paternalism," *The Medical Post,* 1997; 33 (February 11), 34. The Alberta regulations are available from the College. All subsequent quotes from this source. See also *Biomedical Therapy,* 1998; 16(2), 201-202. The reaction to the College's response by Alberta physicians who practiced complementary medicine was strongly negative. Compare Z. P. Rona, "The A-cops strike back," <http://www.wwonline.com/rona/a_cops.htm> (accessed December 1998, no longer available). For comments, York University Centre for Health Studies, *Comple-*

mentary and Alternative Health Practices and Therapies, a Canadian Overview, 1999, pp. 105-107.

21. Medical Profession Amendment Act, 1996, S.A. 1996, c.27, s.2.

22. Regulations available from the College of Physicians and Surgeons of Manitoba.

23. Regulations available from The College of Physicians and Surgeons of Ontario. See also <http://www.cpso.on.ca/articles.asp?ArticleId=874950197> (accessed September 2001). As in Alberta efforts were made in Ontario (1998-1999) to establish legislation that would restrain the College of Physicians and Surgeons from using its disciplinary powers to harass doctors solely because they practice complementary or alternative medicine (see <http://www.life.ca/nl/65/krop.html>, accessed July 1999). The Ontario Policy, albeit with similarities to the Alberta and Manitoba directives, suggests a more liberal attitude. For instance, physicians should be allowed a "reasonable and responsible degree of latitude in the kinds of therapies they offer to their patients. We also believe that patients have every right to seek whatever kind of therapy they want."

24. Available from Board or at <http://www.tsbme.state.tx.us/rules/200.htm> (accessed September 2001).

25. M. Oliver, "MDs Remain Sceptical as Chelation Goes Mainstream in Saskatchewan," *Canadian Medical Association Journal,* 1997; 157, 750-753. *Maclean's,* 1999; 112 (July 12), 50, reports a doctor "under investigation" by the Ontario College of Physicians and Surgeons for practicing chelation therapy.

26. Despite the widespread interest in, and promotion of, complementary/alternative medicine, few questions are raised in nursing. For an exception: Editorial, "Maintaining 'Alternative' Standards," *The Nurse Practitioner,* 1999; 24(5), 16-17; but see also, "Complementary and Alternative Therapies: Role and Responsibilities of the Registered Nurse," *ConceRN,* 1999; 28 (1), 16-18.

27. For general discussion: J. K. Crellin, "Alternative Medicine. Ethical Challenges for the Profession of Pharmacy," in J. M. Humber and R. F. Almeder, *Alternative Medicine and Ethics,* Totowa, NJ: Humana Press, 1998, pp. 197-212. For an "official" statement from British pharmacy: "Society's evidence to Lord's Enquiry into complementary medicine," *Pharmaceutical Journal,* 1999; 263, 740-741.

28. For other resistance to professionalization: H. A. Baer, J. Hays, N. McClendan, N. McGoldrick, and R. Vespucci, "The Holistic Health Movement in the San Francisco Bay Area: Some Preliminary Observations," *Social Science and Medicine,* 1998; 47, 1495-1501.

29. For nineteenth-century water-cure and other aspects of calls for change: S. E. Cayleff, *Wash and Be Healed:* The Water-Cure Movement and Women's Health, Philadelphia, Temple University Press, 1987.

30. This is clear in all countries under consideration, but has been written up most clearly for Britain, e.g., M. Saks, "Professionalism and Health Care," in D. Field and S. Taylor, eds., *Sociological Perspectives on Health, Illness and Health Care,* Oxford: Blackwell Science, 1988, pp. 174-191.

31. Compare S. Cant and U. Sharma, "Demarcation and Transformation Within Homeopathic Knowledge: A Strategy of Professionalization," *Social Science and Medicine,* 1996; 42, 579-588.

32. Despite the changing attitudes there remains skepticism such that many claim that complemetary/alternative medicine still rejects the scientific model. For example, C. Feasby, "Determining Standard of Care in Alternative Contexts," *Health Law Journal,* 1997; 5, 45-65.

33. See Web site of office: <http://nccam.nih.gov> (accessed September 2001). For some background to the politics and the science: M. C. Miles, "Expanding Med ical Horizons: The National Institutes of Health Office of Alternative Medicine," *Knowledge and Society,* 1998; 11, 87-105; also J. H. Young, "The Development of the Office of Alternative Medicine in the National Institutes, 1991-1996," *Bulletin of the History of Medicine,* 1998; 72, 279-282.

34. As an example of discussion in a similar vein, D. Ullman, "Homeopathy and Managed Care: Manageable or Unmanageable," *Journal of Alternative and Complementary Medicine,* 1999; 5, 65-73.

35. For a sense of the importance of increasingly available funding from government resources, at least in the United States, K. Arnold, "Alternative Medicines Gain in Popularity, Merit Closer Scrutiny," *Journal of the National Cancer Institute,* 1999; 91, 1104-1105.

36. J. Esso, B. M. Berman, A. J. Vickers, and K. Linde, "Complementary Medicine and the Cochrane Collaboration," *JAMA,* 1998; 280, 1628-1630.

37. K. Linde, K. Jobst, and J. Panton, "Acupuncture for Chronic Asthma" (Cochrane Review), in: The Cochrane Library, 1998, Issue 3, 2000, Oxford: Update Software.

38. For interesting discussion by British physician D. Black, "The Limitations of Evidence," *Perspectives in Biology and Medicine,* 1998; 42, 1-7. He emphasizes that evidence-based medicine must not be equated with the whole of medicine. S.W. Goodman, "Who Will Challenge Evidence-Based Medicine?" *Journal Royal College of Physicians of London,* 1999; 33, 249-251.

39. See K. G. Sweeney, D. MacAuley, and D. Pereira Gray, "Personal Significance: The Third Dimension," *Lancet,* 1998; 351, 134-136. For background, such volumes as C. Vincent and A. Furnham, *Complementary Medicine: A Research Perspective,* New York: Wiley, 1997.

40. A. Vickers, "Complementary Medicine or Antagonistic Medicine?" *Complementary Therapies in Medicine,* 1999; 7, 125.

41. It is of particular interest that recent surveys of users in the United States and Canada indicate that 42 percent of adults had used some type of alternative care in the past year. For the U.S. survey by Michigan-based consumer research firm InterActive Solutions, see Business Wire Healthwire, January 27, 1998, sponsored by a managed care company, Landmark Healthcare Inc. A few months earlier (August, 1997), a Canadian poll (CTA/Angus Reid) found the same figure.

42. Compare M. Hardey, "Doctors in the House: The Internet As a Source of Lay Health Knowledge and the Challenge to Expertise," *Sociology of Health and Illness,* 1999; 21, 820-835.

43. The reasons listed are taken from a number of surveys: CTV/Angus Reid survey, Canada (1997); J. A. Astin, "Why Patients Use Alternative Medicine: Results of a National Study," *JAMA,* 1998; 279, 1548-1553; for comments, ibid., 1998; 280, 1659-1661; T. J. Kaptchuk and D. M. Eisenberg, "The Persuasive Appeal of Alter-

native Medicine," *Annals of Internal Medicine,* 1998; 129, 1061-1065. (The authors argue for many similarities between conventional and complementary/alternative medicine.) A recent review with reference to the British scene: C. Vincent and A. Furnham, "Complementary Medicine: State of the Evidence," *Journal of the Royal Society of Medicine,* 1999; 92, 170-177. E. Ernst, K. L. Resch, and S. Hill, "Do Complementary Practitioners Have a Better Bedside Manner Than Physicians?" *Journal of the Royal Society of Medicine* 1997; 90, 118-119. Specifically on health food stores, B. C. Eliason, J. Kruger, D. Mark, and D.N. Rasmann, "Dietary Supplement Users: Demographics, Product Use, and Medical System Interaction," *Journal of the American Board of Family Practitioners,* 1997; 10, 265-267, 271.

44. Compare C. B. Cohen, S. E. Wheeler, D. A. Scott, B. S. Edwards, P. Lusk, and the Anglican Working Group in Bioethics, "Prayer As Therapy: A Challenge to Both Religious Belief and Professional Ethics," *Hastings Center Report,* 2000; May-June, 40-47; A. Sheikh, "Religion, Health and Suffering," *Journal of the Royal Society of Medicine,* 1999; 92, 600-601. Perhaps greatest interest is emerging in nursing. See, too, R.C. Fuller, *Alternative Medicine and American Religious Life,* New York: Oxford University Press, 1989.

45. This leads to a growing literature along the lines of J. Krohn and F. Taylor, *Finding the Right Cure: Making Informed Choices About Conventional and Alternative Medicine,* Point Roberts: Hartley and Marks, 1998.

46. European Commission, *Cost Action B4 Unconventional Medicine,* Luxembourg: Office for Official Publications of the European Communities, 1999, p. 39.

47. This is documented in many ways, e.g., R. Herzlinger, *Market-Driven Health Care: Who Wins, Who Loses in the Transformation of America's Largest Service Industry,* Reading, PA: Addison-Wesley, 1997.

Chapter 3

Changing the Health Care Paradigm?

INTRODUCTION

Scrutinies of complementary/alternative medicine in Western countries coincide with widespread concerns over the rising costs of mainstream health care, and with changes in its administration and delivery. Although these changes have been initiated largely by economic problems, much agreement exists that reform is needed anyway to improve the overall quality of health care. Calls exist on both sides of the Atlantic to "rebalance" the roles of hospital and community services. Also raised is the question, Will complementary/alternative medicine contribute to overall change? At present, as already noted, most of its practitioners seem more concerned with reform within their field rather than in health care as a whole. In fact, arguments that complementary/alternative medicine can make a real change in health care come more from its grassroots support than from its practitioners. Indeed some commentators suggest that complementary/alternative care—as part of the consumer movement with emphasis on wellness—has already had an impact. For instance, its recent beneficial role in bringing about a greater spirit of self-criticism within the health and social-service professions, as well as wider assertiveness and activism among the public, has been noted by an authority on the history of the British National Health Service:

> The charismatic voices of Illich, Foucault, the Neo-Marxists, and the anti-psychiatry movement, together with the new-found confidence within complementary medicine, contributed to a new dynamic and plurality of thinking about medicine that proved capable of sustaining itself into the 1990s as a constructive force.[1]

In this chapter, with its question mark about change in the health care paradigm, we look at a range of issues relevant both to whether a significant change will take place and to matters of professionalism. For instance, health care values, economics, ideologies, the extent to which people are taking greater responsibility for their own health, the need of choices for patients, and other issues are raised constantly by practitioners, users of complementary/alternative medicine, and commentators.[2] Among the questions this raises is, How proactive should complementary/alternative practitioners be in demanding reform in their own field and in health care in general?

VALUES IN HEALTH CARE

Although many people believe that improving the status quo—always a professional responsibility—is only to be done through research on therapies, other ways of contributing to health care exist, many suited to a practitioner's everyday professional practice. A particular issue today is to raise questions about the place of values in health care. What values should practitioners protect? There is a growing concern that "traditional" values (meaning, for example, compassion, caring, integrity) are being pushed to one side, or lost amid changes in mainstream health care. Questions being asked are: What basic values must be preserved? Do patients have the same values as practitioners? What are professional values and, if they clash with institutional values, which should take precedence? Do complementary/alternative and conventional practitioners have the same values? While we now offer some brief general remarks on these matters, other relevant discussion appears in Part II.

First, what exactly do we mean by values? The term, used in a variety of contexts (e.g., aesthetic values, economic values, religious values), indicates what is felt to be important or to be cherished, what has worth, what is desired. The following "definitions" capture general meanings.

1. *Values,* when used without any other defining term (such as economic values) refer to what is morally good (moral values), such as compassion or respecting the best interests of others. Moral values are embodied in moral *principles,* which refer to actions that are not only right or obligatory, but are also generally accepted as being universally held within a society (e.g., principles of justice and beneficence).

2. *Individual or personal values* may well be positive ideals, but are not necessarily morally good. They can range from wanting certain material possessions, such as an expensive car or house (perhaps linked to demands for high incomes from one's profession) to the values associated with particular religious groups, such as the avoidance of blood transfusions by Jehovah's Witnesses. Clearly, such values can vary significantly from individual to individual.

3. *Professional values,* commonly embodied in codes of ethics, are those accepted by the profession. They normally embrace moral values. Dilemmas may well arise when individual values (e.g., derived from religious teachings) and professional values clash.[3]

These definitions are not mutually exclusive; justice, for instance, fits into all three categories.

More specifically, what values are associated particularly with health care? Here, we can only give a brief response. A convenient, if arbitrary, place to start is the list of values emerging from an Ethics Working Group that was formed as part of President Clinton's 1993-1994 campaign for health care reform in the United States. Although tensions and differences of opinion existed within the Group, it established a list of values and principles (relevant to the health care systems and to individual practitioners) that deserve the attention of any practitioner. Indeed, the list challenges individuals to examine their own values and their responsibilities in health care systems as a whole. First, the Group agreed that "health care is of fundamental moral importance because it protects our opportunity to pursue life goals, reduces our pain and suffering, prevents premature loss of life, and provides information needed to plan our lives." Given this, the Group stated that health care must embrace the following values:[4]

1. *Caring for all.* Because health care is a fundamental good, the moral ideals of justice, equality, and community require that the health care system provides: universal access, comprehensive benefits, equal benefits, fair burdens, and generational solidarity.

2. *Making the system work.* The health care system must allocate wisely, treat effectively, ensure quality, and manage efficiently.

Controlling costs without unduly compromising quality is a moral, not just an economic imperative.

3. *Choice and responsibility.* The health care system must respect the choices appropriately left to patients or providers, encourage personal responsibility, and protect professional integrity, while ensuring accountability through fair procedures.

It is noteworthy that, for various reasons, the Clinton Group presented their list of values as if they were independent concepts, that is without justifying them on the basis of such universal principles as justice and equality. In fact, without underlying theory or justification, it can be difficult to prioritize values in particular situations; for example, is a society's health care responsibilities—in the context of scarce resources—to the young the same as those to the elderly?

Complementary/alternative practitioners will undoubtedly accept these values, but regret that they are applied unevenly. The extent to which this unevenness will change is an issue for each practitioner. For instance, are the values relevant beyond the needs of individual patients such that the practitioners should lobby for improved health care within their communities, or even within society at large? Indeed, should the values of all health care practitioners embrace being proactive in responding to community/social needs? We also ask, How open should practitioners be about their values? How many practitioners make their values clear to all patients? Is there, for instance, a responsibility to indicate the limitations of one's practice? While such matters are for individual practitioners to decide, their relevance to health reform in general and to professionalism must be constantly borne in mind.

ECONOMIC ISSUES

The commercial settings in which so much complementary/alternative medicine takes place raise questions about and clashes between values. For instance, concerns are often raised that rampant commercialism and mass marketing of products (e.g., Chinese herbs) push aside the traditional experiences and ways of using herbs, and reshape modern usage. In addition, many in the world of growing and processing herbs see themselves, not surprisingly, as part of the agricultural/horticultural/manufacturing industries, rather than of health care. Differences between business and health care ethics becomes an issue. Although common ground exists—both are applied moral ethics—most views focus on a significant difference in basic premises. A common view is that business ethics center solely on the need to maximize profits, albeit with a sense that this, through a trickle down effect, benefits society at large. Health care ethics, on the other hand, although not ignoring communities, constantly raises concerns about how to serve the best interests of individuals, individuals whose responses to health and illness can vary significantly. Business, in general, only serves individuals if their needs fit into a large group.

This lack of attention to individuals leads AIDS organizations, for example, to suggest that business has no social concerns, and that the "cost of dietary supplements be reviewed by regulatory agencies."[5] In lobbying for reform, various constituencies raise additional ethical concerns about complementary/alternative practitioners selling preparations, from their own offices or dispensaries, at inflated prices. On the other hand, arguments that this allows practitioners some control over consistent quality of products may well be valid (compare Quality and Standardization of Preparations in Chapter 4).

Practitioners of complementary/alternative medicine face other potential ethical issues that center on costs such as fees, phone call consultations, etc., all of which can be addressed through information available in waiting rooms and through fully informed consent. Practitioners must also make clear treatment goals and practice boundaries to preempt suspicions of improprieties such as "high costs" of "nonbeneficial" treatment. For instance, in the Canadian case of Dr. Krop, already noted, the College of Physicians and Surgeons of Ontario wrote in a news release: "The [College] Committee is aware of substantial sums expended by [patients] . . . and is concerned about the potential hardships of such expenditures. Recommendations for lifestyle changes—such as elimination of a wide variety of foods from the diet, rigid adherence to a variety of 'desensitizing' regimens, and the recommendation to quit a job and undergo sauna treatment— pose additional costs. In the Committee's view, if unjustified, these constitute a form of harm."[6]

Broader economic issues also attract attention. One is public demand for much wider insurance coverage, private or national, as the high costs of complementary/alternative medicine are not affordable by all.[7] At present in the United States, private coverage, which became much more widespread in the 1990s, is variable, and, of course, there is no national health system as there is in, say, Britain and Canada.[8] Economic barriers violate such health care values as universal access, individual choice, and justice—as users commonly point out—especially for those (e.g., sufferers from AIDS) who see complementary/alternative care as making a major contribution to quality of life.

In the context of costs of complementary/alternative care and insurance, many ask whether public funds should be used to reduce costs, bearing in mind consumer demand. The belief of many Canadians (1997) that government health care plans should cover complementary/alternative care resonates with 67 percent of U.S. citizens surveyed in 1998 who indicated that the availability of alternative care is an important factor in choosing a health care plan.[9] Of course, this raises such questions as whether, if public funds are used, should they only be for proven treatments? After all, health care constantly has to deal with the ethics of allocating scarce resources.

There are also demands to control high costs due to expensive government bureaucracy and inefficiency. Critiques—from those who, through experience, are genuinely frustrated with contradictions and inconsistencies in government, and from those whose personal ideologies stem from antigovernment, anti-big business and antiscience views—pinpoint "insurmountable barriers" for small businesses. They say, too, that bureaucracy will likely become more costly if new regulatory processes are put in place and, in consequence, put small companies out of business, a development that will curb freedom of choice.[10]

One economic argument for change in the health care paradigm is that complementary/alternative medicine (especially acupuncture, chiropractic and homeopathy) can reduce the overall costs of health care through both treatment and prevention. Unfortunately, evidence on cost-benefits of treatments provides mixed conclusions over whether this is so. For instance, vigorous disagreement exists over the results of studies on the economic benefits of chiropractic for low back pain.[11] Further, the role in prevention is questioned on the grounds that the preventive thrusts of complementary/alternative medicine are poorly, if at all, integrated with regular public health campaigns to reduce, for example, heart disease and cervical cancer. Presently, although we now have accepted methodologies for cost-benefit analysis, there is still little incontrovertible evidence to challenge such statements as "there is no hard evidence [despite the use of fewer tests and lower treatment costs] to support the notion that complementary medicine is cost-beneficial, and further trials are necessary."[12]

A further point about public calls for change merits notice here, since it raises further concerns over safety, fairness and justice. It is about the natural health products and pharmaceuticals available for purchase via the Internet. Consumers can acquire items that are unavailable or banned in their own country. For instance, with regard to Canada, one commentator stated (1998) that a U.S. company "has 858 products, 42 percent of which cannot legally be sold in Canada."[13] Economic losses to Canadian industry are often highlighted, along with costs to patients and worries about quality and safety. On these latter grounds, questions arise whether complementary/alternative practitioners should encourage the public to import such products from another country, even if permitted to do so for "personal use," unless they are able to evaluate safety and quality.[14] Clearly, professional responsibility and leadership is needed in critically debating many economic issues.

ANTIMEDICINE/ANTISCIENCE, ANTIGOVERNMENT, ANTI-BIG BUSINESS

It is often said that calls for a paradigm shift in health care are directly related to dissatisfaction with mainstream medicine. Dissatisfaction may be directed toward health care systems, treatments, or physicians. Complaints about the latter are well known and one example will suffice in which physicians were said to ignore patients with fibromyalgia. "When you go to a doctor now, to get a consultation or to even get a doctor, they will first come into the room and ask you flat out if you have fibromyalgia chronic fatigue. If you say yes, they tell you on the spot 'I have the right not to accept you as a patient.' [Then they refuse a consultation and tell you] to go to the walk-in clinics."[15]

However, the overall impact of such episodes for fostering the growth of complementary/alternative medicine is not altogether clear. In Canada, for example, according to a 1997 poll, relatively few users indicate that a main reason for utilizing alternative medicine is because they "don't trust modern medicine and practices."[16] And a 1999 U.S. study indicated that not all users of complementary/alternative medicine had lost faith in science—51 percent claimed that scientific reports are more important than testimonials, word-of-mouth reports, and a long history of usage.[17] On the other hand, U.K. studies (1995 and 1997) on attitudes to science and medicine among patients attending an osteopath, homeopath, acupuncturist or a regular general practitioner revealed, not surprisingly, more positive attitudes toward "orthodox medicine" among those visiting the GP. Users of complementary/alternative care attached importance to psychological factors though this was not consistent for all modalities.[18] There is no way of knowing whether or not an apparently high level of trust in mainstream physicians owes at least something to the way the medical profession has been responding, in recent years, to societal concerns about physician insensitivity. After all, psychosocial care, medical communication, ethics, and the humanities have gained a formal place in medical education. However, the overall impact is slow, and criticism of poor communication continues, as do views that professional values can be self-serving and often fail to protect the public from poor practices.[19]

Even if the growth of interest in complementary/alternative medicine is prompted less by a mistrust of physicians than is sometimes supposed, concerns over many aspects of the science of medicine and medical technology fuel calls for a new health care paradigm (compare also As a Scientist in Chapter 7). Worries over, for example, over-reliance on "laboratory-produced synthetic" medicines and their side effects—often reinforced by the environment movement—are conspicuous. Increasingly, in recent years, the presumed safety of "natural" products has been contrasted with synthetics and other "doctor-induced" diseases. Many consider that statistics on, for example, the dangers of prescription drugs (e.g., 106,000 deaths from adverse drug reactions in U.S. hospitals in 1994) support the continuing influence of Ivan Illich, whose *Medical Nemesis* (1967) argues that Western medicine has become a major threat to health.[20] When mainstream physicians dismiss such views as alarmist or as "emotional" responses, they need to understand deep-seated fears of side effects. Such fears are fed in many ways, including by complementary/alternative practitioners who, when failing to offer patients balanced perspectives, may not be providing optimum quality care. For instance, background information and perspective might need to be given on such lay views as "a great deal of synthetics, especially those synthetics used to beat cancer, are toxic. Chemotherapy, for example, involves a mustard gas that was used on the battlefield to kill people during World War I. How can we kill selectively that way: kill cancer and spare the healthy one?"[21]

The above concerns are compounded by criticisms of the way science is applied and administered by government agencies. Although some of the criticism—from redundant government scientists—may not be without bias, "insider" opinions reinforce public suspicions about the integrity of public (and private) institutions, the gulf between administrators and scientists, the "state of rot" from ineffective leadership and long-range planning, and the limited scientific, medical, and even regulatory knowledge among administrators.[22] Especially noticeable are worries—among a broad sweep of political scientists and advocates of complementary/alternative medicine—about collusion between government and "big" business. Particular cause de cèlébres such as side effects of tryptophan (see Box 3.1) foster deep suspicions.

BOX 3.1. Concerns Over Science: Tryptophan

Various "episodes" have exacerbated public suspicions of science in recent years. Proponents of complementary/alternative medicine often raise queries about the safety of tryptophan and nifedepine. The continuing influence of the tryptophan toxicity episode in many countries was highlighted before the Canadian House of Commons Standing Committee on Health in 1998:

> Some 10 or 12 years ago [tryptophan, marketed as a dietary supplement for insomnia, depression and other conditions] was banned from the marketplace because of a contaminant by a Japanese manufacturer. The contaminant was isolated and removed, but all the tryptophan was banned. That's akin to two or three of you people going and having supper at [one] local restaurant and getting sick and the health authorities close down all the restaurants in the national capital region. . . .
> Interestingly, the time was crucial, because Prozac was coming on the marketplace at around the same time, acting similarly to tryptophan. The opportunity was there [and taken] to ban the competition to Prozac. There are people who think that in fact the contaminant was seeded; it wasn't part of the manufacturing process at all.*

This interpretation is in line with a generally accepted view which coupled with the particular sensitivity of some people, contaminants in tryptophan were the cause of many serious cases (including deaths) of eosinophilia-myalgia

(continued)

(continued)

syndrome. However, what is not considered are the concerns of scientists that tryptophan may not be manufactured commercially free of toxic contaminants. Moreover, doubts still exist over the safety of tryptophan itself.**

---

*House of Common Standing Committee on Health Minutes, February 25, 1998, p. 18.

**See FDA talk paper, "Impurities Confirmed in Dietary Supplements 5-Hydroxy-L-Tryptophan," August, 1998, <http://vm.cfsan.fda.gov/n/tp5htp.html>, House of Commons Standing Committee on Health Minutes, February 25, 1998, p. 19.

Biases

The dissatisfaction and calls for change outlined so far embrace particular points of view and special interests. This should prompt all practitioners to look for pervasive biases in themselves as well as in their own disciplines. These can be difficult to uncover. As an example, the 1998 study, "Conflict of Interest in the Debate over Calcium-Channel Antagonists,"[23] has attracted much attention. On reviewing studies on antagonists, it found that authors who supported the use of calcium channel antagonists were significantly more likely, than "neutral" or "critical" authors, to have financial relationships with manufacturers of the medicines or other pharmaceutical companies. This led one lay observer to find difficulty with the "whole theory about research. What they have here is science, theoretically double-blind science, which actually supports the drug product in the end."[24]

Biases among editors on what gets published raise further issues. For instance, the editors of the *Journal of the American Medical Association* ranked alternative medicine sixty-eight out of seventy-three topics in order of priority, whereas readers ranked it number seven.[25] And, of course, language barriers—the bulk of research on herbs is published in non-English language journals—can have the same effect as a bias.

TWO CULTURES, BELIEFS ABOUT DISEASE, HOLISM, AND HEALTH

In this section we comment on some interrelated matters, on ideologies, on beliefs about disease, on concepts of health and on attitudes as they impinge on current practices and matters of professionalism. In doing so, we remind readers that understanding different beliefs and concepts and interpreting data is part of a systematic approach to an ethical dilemma, and to quality of care. In fact, much uncertainty in health care arises from different interpretations of concepts, of patients' stories, of test results, and much more. We might add that hermeneutics, the philosopher's term for the systematic study of interpretation, is not inappropriate to describe how a practitioner approaches decision making when searching for the best care for a patient.[26]

Two Cultures

Amid calls for changes in the current health care paradigm on both sides of the Atlantic and elsewhere, unease, if not confrontation, exists between two cultures in health care or, as often expressed, two worldviews, two ways of looking at or interpreting "facts." A report on a 1998 controversy about vitamin B_6 characterized sharp dichotomies of opinion. The British government proposed, because of a perceived safety hazard, that 10 mg should be the upper dosage limit allowed for the general sale of vitamin B_6 as a "dietary supplement." A furor of protest emerged from the estimated "three million Britons who take daily doses up to 200 mg." The pros and cons against the sale of large doses as a safe dietary supplement were described as two cultures: the "culture gap could not be wider."[27] The defining characteristics of the two cultures depend somewhat on the observer; however, generally speaking, one culture includes those who look to change (or to "reform") health care to a more natural way, who perhaps see the spiritual and physical worlds as manifestations of a single life force—i.e., mind, body, and spirit are inseparable. The other culture sees conventional medicine as resting on science, hence the terms biomedicine or scientific medicine.

Of course, the "real" world is somewhat more complex than just two polarized cultures, for each embraces a spectrum of opinions about the worlds of science and of nonscience, just as different opinions can be found among practitioners offering the same therapy.[28] Understanding different attitudes toward the two cultures and the concepts, beliefs and rationales found within each is professionally important, if only as a way of fostering effective communication through a better understanding of individual patients (see As a Communicator, in Chapter 7).[29] Here we offer some introductory notes beginning with ideologies.

Lay Ideologies and Beliefs About Disease

The term ideology (some prefer the term mind-set) can be confusing because of the various ways it is employed in everyday use. However, ideologies can be said to exist as *strongly held beliefs* or strong commitments to an idea or a teaching, or to a cluster of closely related ideas. While this can mean a commitment to what others consider an evident falsity, or a lack of openness to conflicting ideas or interpretations, it must not be dismissed without careful evaluation.

Complementary/alternative care is commonly dismissed as being based on ideologies rather than sound observation. Although this often reflects a lack of understanding on the part of a critic, it should alert its practitioners to examine critically the basic premises that underpin their practice. For instance, some may promote environmental factors as "poisoning" bodily systems; although at times unquestionably true, the question needs to be asked: Is the concept fostered as much by a long history of beliefs in Western culture—e.g., the innate dangers of civilization, of urban living, of violating nature, and the need to live the "right way"—as by firm scientific data?[30] Complementary/alternative practitioners also need to respond to the criticism that they often accept uncritically, at least more so than physicians, popular beliefs. This criticism, however, may overlook the empirical basis of many beliefs, and that they are often viewed as "common sense," meaning reliance on long-standing everyday experiences and the observations of others.

Although this is not the place for a detailed discussion on popular beliefs, a few notes are a reminder, especially to physicians, of this important aspect of health care. Theories of disease over time can be broadly grouped into two, albeit not mutually exclusive, categories: (1) changes within the body, and (2) conditions linked to "outside" or "environmental" factors. Internal changes may be associated with the long-standing, still influential concept of vitalism, often expressed today in terms of life forces or energy medicine. Notions of vitalism remain pervasive in long-standing medical traditions (e.g., traditional Chinese medicine), as well as in such practices as homeopathy and magnet therapy. Although few scientists currently consider notions about imbalances of vital forces as a serious challenge to conventional physiological theories, there are those who believe that we are moving toward a new "energy" paradigm in medical science—a shift from almost complete emphasis on biochemistry to the study of the physical properties of matter.

Internal bodily changes are also spoken of nowadays in terms of toxemia ("autointoxication," "accumulation of waste matter," and so on), or as the result of the presence of a dangerous "build-up" of free radicals that contribute to ageing and degeneration (a view increasingly supported by science.) Such toxemia concepts contribute to a widespread promotion, especially within much complementary/alternative health care, of detoxification regimens. A popular concept, too, is that the body has a natural tendency to maintain and heal itself, and that health care should aim to encourage, not interfere, with this. The innate ability of the body to cure itself is part of the notion of restoring imbalance (of, for instance, vital energy), within the body so as to attain good health. Imbalance, it is said, can be reflected in, for example, constipation, diarrhea, fevers or headaches, which are signs that toxins exist in the bloodstream, and, in the cases of diarrhea and fever, are being eliminated.[31] Indeed, so widespread is the interest in balance that some consider searching for the right balance in life—perhaps spiritual needs—is instinctive, and leads many to explore complementary/alternative therapies.[32]

Disease agents that act from outside the body include "germs" (in complementary/alternative medicine, candida and "animalcules" are often diagnosed) and the influence of the weather, of draughts, of getting one's feet wet. Some see these ideas as akin to the concepts of cold, heat, wind, and damp in traditional Chinese medicine. Other external factors (e.g., toxins such as PCBs, lead, and mercury) and radiation (e.g., radon) received increasing attention in the 1980s and 1990s, and have also drawn on concepts of rebalancing, for instance, if the immune system has been "poisoned."

Any consideration of patients and their nonconventional beliefs may include assessing whether the beliefs are part of a spectrum of dissenting, nonmainstream views. Relevant to this are the findings of a U.S. study that identified the emergence of a group of individuals (estimated to be 24 percent of U.S. adults), who have been called "cultural creatives."[33] They contrast with "traditionalists" (who are conservative and believe in the nostalgic image of small American towns) and "modernists" (who place high value on personal success, consumerism, materialism, and technological rationality). The attitudes or values of the cultural creatives include profeminism, holism, concerns over the environment, and the view that nature is sacred. Many cultural creatives also wish to have more control or "empowerment" in their health care and are recognized as a "core market for psychotherapy, alternative health care, and natural foods."

Ideologies Within Science and Medicine

Many people see ideologies in complementary/alternative, but not in mainstream medicine. They see the latter as based only on "fact," on observing and responding to observable/measurable pathology in organs, tissues, or body fluids. This approach prompts concerns that conventional medicine is narrow in focus. Physicians are chastized for an ideology of "reductionism" when this is taken to mean seeing illness, at least in principle, in terms of physical or biochemical changes alone (associated with laboratory investigations and medical technology), in contrast to seeing it in terms of interaction of body, mind, and spirit.

In fact, the term reductionism is best reserved as a benchmark of the scientific method, as a research strategy to isolate and investigate separately the many variables in, say, a biological system. Although many scientists see it as a research strategy only—a very successful one—concerns exist about its dominance in investigating natural phenomenon. Within complementary/alternative medicine many argue that a "holistic science" approach should be taken that emphasizes the importance of investigating ecological and other contexts. Physicians, on the other hand, may argue that reductionism in medicine is merely a strategy on how best to approach an illness in which variables are isolated and studied, but with an appreciation that the whole can be more than the sum of the parts. Even so, criticisms that physicians view reductionism as an ultimate strategy and goal rather than one approach to diagnosis and treatment can be valid.[34] There are, too, concerns that reductionism will be fostered by the growing use of computerized databases—that provide both "diagnoses" and treatment regimens. This also applies to complementary/alternative practices (e.g., in herbal medicine and homeopathy), and can obviously become a professional issue if it reshapes practices.[35]

It is appropriate to add that reductionism in medicine became increasingly an issue with the nineteenth-century trend to see science as a "central dogma" in the pursuit of truth. In remaining the prevailing ideology, it commonly escapes critical appraisal such that biases in research, as we noted over calcium-channel antagonists, are slow in being uncovered. We cannot explore here the common ideology that science produces truth, beyond emphasizing the need for humility every time a scientific idea is debunked. New interpretations of existing data come and go, sometimes due to selective mining of information (e.g., the heretical view (in 2000) that atherosclerosis is linked less to high intake of saturated fatty acids than to infectious disease).

Many users of complementary/alternative medicine see science as an "ideological mind-set" that fosters arrogance.[36] This extends to dismissing the possibility that outsiders to the profession can make contributions to new knowledge. Examples range from the story of *Lorenzo's Oil* (see Box 3.2), to negative "attitudes" toward micronutrient supplements among U.S. academic physicians. It has been shown that physicians, in uncritically rejecting "outside" opinions that high doses of vitamins or minerals are toxic, reveal an inbuilt bias.[37] It is, too, such a scientific mind-set that often defines "heresies" found within medicine, including, of course, complementary/alternative medicine.[38] Clearly this adds to the difficulties of integration.

BOX 3.2. Lorenzo's Oil and Hollywood

Lorenzo's Oil, a 1992 movie, is based on a true story that took place between 1884 and 1887. When Augusta and Michaela Odone learned that their five-year-old child had a rare terminal disease, adrenoleukodystrophy, they set out on a mission to find a cure using the scientific method. In so doing, they collided with doctors, scientists and support groups who felt the search was not their job. The oil has proved disappointing in terms of cure, but for pertinent comments on its role in affecting the course of the condition appeared in the Odone's "More on Lorenzo's Oil," *New England Journal of Medicine,* 1994; 330, 1904.

Attitudes

Any consideration of beliefs and ideologies must also look at "attitudes." Like ideologies, attitudes can be strongly held, but generally they are understood as being less rigid and more open to change. For instance, the attitude of many users of natural health products is that, while evidence of effectiveness of a product may be limited and uncertain (or the product may be a fad), it is prudent to try it until other information becomes available.[39]

Quality health care must recognize the existence of a kaleidoscope of attitudes and beliefs from, for example, aboriginal, ayurvedic, traditional Chinese medicine, and other traditions, to specific religious prohibitions such as blood transfusions for Jehovah's Witnesses or pork insulin for Jews. A practitioner's attitudes can also be an important consideration. In our discussion on practitioner as communicator (see Chapter 7), we notice that practitioners' attitudes toward patients can be reflected in their general demeanor (nonverbal behavior) and in casual "off-the-cuff" remarks.

Holism and Health

The concept of holism, which some say has been hijacked by complementary/alternative medicine, has many shades of meaning and much misuse in health care.[40] Interestingly, the concept—most generally referring to all aspects of a patient's physical and mental health—is not as recent as often supposed. It has appeared in different guises many times in the twentieth century, commonly arising from concerns about what are seen as reductionist trends in mainstream medicine already noted.[41]

The current preoccupation with holism is driven by various social currents. It is partly a response to reductionism and to the view that scientific explanation must be expanded to embrace considerations such as holistic science and chaos theory, as physicians sometimes debate.[42] There is, too, a new readiness to explore spiritual needs, which, as noted earlier, often leads to interest in the New Age eclecticism of ideas that cover complementary/alternative practices and concepts such as balance within the body and between the body and the environment. It is not surprising that a 1998 study showed that homeopathic patients, in endorsing central tenets of the practice, believed not only in the treatment of the whole person, but also—more strongly than the patients of a general practitioner—in the self-healing power of the body.[43]

Nowadays, holism is also commonly viewed as summarizing the "modern" definition of health stemming from the World Health Organization. This sees health as a state of complete physical, mental and social well-being, and not merely the absence of physical illness, which is another way of describing "wellness," the search for which is now widespread. In contrast, the concept of holism is sometimes, confusingly, appropriated for specific approaches within health care. For example, holism may refer to a practice such as acupuncture because of its unitary theory of balancing yin and yang, to an empathic understanding of patients, to making sure there is sufficient time in a consultancy so that patients do not feel pressured, or to ensuring that hope is not extinguished (see Efficacy, Effectiveness, and Placebos, in Chapter 4). Holism is even used to describe such nonmainstream practices as colonic hydrotherapy.[44]

Clearly, there is a need to examine critically the meanings given to holism, and the attacks on mainstream medicine for not being holistic. Many physicians argue that their practice—perhaps consciously based on biopsychosocial care—*is* holistic, for they define it as paying attention to all aspects of a patient's mental and physical health. Indeed, some see their holistic approach as "healing" (see As a Healer, in Chapter 7). These physicians (and nurses with the same mind-set) may belong to holistic medical and nursing organizations with such goals as:

1. responding to a person as a whole within their environment and seeing that person as mind, body, and spirit;
2. being open to a wide range of approaches, not only drugs and surgery, but also education, communication, self-help, and complementary therapies;
3. returning power and responsibility to patients wherever appropriate, encouraging self-awareness and capacity for self-healing; and
4. recognizing that the carer is also a whole person, needing care, support, and the chance to develop and grow.[45]

Some "holistic" physicians critique holism in complementary/alternative care along the lines of M. Baum in "What Is Holism?"[46] Although not unsupportive of the goals just outlined, he writes that the word "holistic" is another example of "debasing the currency of our language . . . to prop up primitive and *closed* belief systems." He criticizes the holism of complementary/alternative medicine as "a purely metaphysical construct where the mind, body and spirit are bound together by vital forces or energy fields. . . . [T]his vital force, these paranormal energy fields, are not open to the experimental method of study and, therefore, have to be considered a surrogate for faith whose popularity increases in our fin de siècle society." Of course, many complementary/alternative practitioners take issue with any dismissal of vitalistic or metaphysical concepts to explain holism. They believe there is much empirical data to support the concept and often cite the healing ceremonies and teachings of aboriginal peoples, which can be expressed as "healing through the four fundamental components of the human being, which are spirit, emotion, body and mind."[47]

In the context of our remarks it would be wrong to say that all complementary/alternative practitioners—past or present—practice holistically in the sense of paying specific attention to mind and spirit as well as physical ills. As J. Stone and J. Matthews have written:

> Contrary to the rhetoric, we cannot assume that all therapists do work in a patient-centred way. Complementary medicine has its fair share of autocratic, domineering practitioners. Nor do all practitioners adopt a holistic approach. Many therapists adopt a multi-therapeutic approach and wander into areas in which they are less qualified to treat patients. There is thus a discrepancy between how practitioners are actually practising and what their codes of ethics prescribe.[48]

The authors indicate that, despite perhaps a unitary theory (e.g., vitalism), a patient may well feel the same sense of reductionism that is at the centre of much criticism of mainstream care. In other words, complementary/alternative modalities may be seen as stripped down to be alternative *medications* alone. Moreover, the rapid growth in popularity of, say, herbal medicine and homeopathy has encouraged notions that "a pill will cure the problem." Nutrition stores, pharmacies and countless advocacy writings foster this by categorizing specific remedies for specific ailments or symptoms. There are, too, such enigmatic episodes in the history of complementary/alternative care as the success of Mahlon Locke, the Canadian physician who acquired in the 1930s a tremendous reputation for his treatment, popularly known as toe-twisting, of arthritis and other ailments (see Box 3.3). His story raises general questions about the role of faith and the importance of the placebo effect in health care considered later.

Our remarks in this section, as said, underscore the importance of practitioners critically evaluating the concept of holism and its role in their practice. In this context, we make one other point. Given the justified unhappiness many have with the looseness of the term holism, it must be said that the fluidity of the meanings attached to it may be a significant aspect of health care. After all, it allows individuals to be comfortable with their own meaning of the term as well as to find like-minded practitionerswho who will work with them. Indeed, this

---

BOX 3.3. Dr. Mahlon Locke—Hardly Holistic Care?

A noteworthy study of Mahlon Locke merits comment in relation to nonholistic care. Practicing an impersonal therapy, the Canadian physician acquired in the 1930s an enormous following for his treatment of arthritis (and other ailments) popularly known as toe-twisting.* At the height of his fame Locke would seat himself, at the beginning of each treatment session, in a swivel chair at the center of the yard while patients waited in a dozen or more lines around him, like spokes radiating from the hub of a wheel. Sufferey reached Locke's chair. With only a cursory glance, he would twist the feet in front of him, perhaps offer a few words of advice, and then spin on to the next patient.

Clow, in looking at patients' responses, suggests several reasons for his success. One must not forget he was a licensed medical practitioner, and his practice could be seen as "scientific." At the same time some saw him with the persona of a wise country doctor and others as a miracle worker. His success undoubtedly owed much to popular stories about him. Patients swapped stories, talked about their illnesses; about their experiences. One eyewitness report stated:

> Outside patients—some twelve hundred of them—were assembling in the pavilion for their afternoon treatments and while they waited for him to take an hour's needed rest, they sang and laughed and joked.*

---

*B. Clow, "'Swapping Grief': The Role of the Laity in Alternative Medical Encounters," *Journal of History of Medicine and Allied Sciences*, 1997; 52, 175-201.

---

fits with the view that holistic care should be seen as a social/therapeutic relationship, rather than as "medical management."

INTEGRATION

One purpose of Chapter 3 ("Changing the Health Care Paradigm?") is to prompt specific consideration of professional responsibilities in connection with integration. After all, many hopes exist for some formal level of integration or collaboration between complementary/alternative and mainstream medicine. However, many of our comments so far—e.g., on anticomplementary/alternative Web sites, such as Quackwatch, on two cultures and on ideologies—all suggest that relatively little common ground exists between mainstream and complementary/alternative medicine. Certainly, many commentators consider that boundaries are firm and that any real integration is very unlikely, except where there are special circumstances, as in Cuba or in China and Japan.[49] Contrarily, others believe a real change has already started.[50] Indeed, many physicians incorporate certain modalities into their practices or refer patients to complementary/alternative practitioners.[51] Furthermore, growing numbers of hospitals offer or link with complementary/alternative care in one way or another. Also, challenges to traditional roles and to medicine's position at the top of the hierarchy of the health professions, as well as changing professional boundaries within, say, the nursing and pharmacy professions, are seen as signs of changes to come.

Given the above trends, it is not surprising that discussions on integrating complementary/alternative medicine into mainstream medicine are now commonplace beyond the establishment of wellness centers with office space for both regular and complementary/alternative practitioners. In 1998, W. B. Jonas said that "today, the overwhelming effort is towards attempts at 'integrating' alternative practices into mainstream."[52] Ethicists, too, see some form of integration as respect for patient autonomy.[53] Certainly, conspicuous features emerged in the late 1990s, ranging from the Foundation for Integrated Medicine in Britain, founded (1997) by the Prince of Wales, to publications with such titles as *Integrative Medicine: Integrating Conventional and Alternative Medicine* (Volume 1, 1998). Further, we have noted the views of at least some complementary/alternative practitioners that integration may well improve their own professional standing. However, this is problematic for other practitioners who see a real risk of eventually losing the advantages of diversity and choice that now exist for patients.[54]

Calls for integration commonly pinpoint frustrations with the limitations of conventional medicine. Specific concerns arise over possible incompatibilities between complementary therapies (especially herbs) and prescription medications. Time and time again, commentators emphasize high numbers (e.g., 15 million U.S. adults) at risk for potential adverse interactions involving prescription medications and herbs or high dose vitamin supplements; furthermore, innumerable patients (in 1997 around 40 percent in the United States) fail to disclose their use of alternative therapies to physicians, though this may well be changing.[55] Overall, an evident desire prevails on the part of many people to harness the best quality-of-life teachings offered by complementary/alternative care with the best of medical science.[56]

Policy discussions on integration often focus on the complementary/alternative modalities or practices that are "appropriate" for mainstream medicine to consider, on the different views about appropriate levels of integration, and on the various approaches or "models" of integration.[57] We indicate some of the issues on three areas of discussion only: (1) selective incorporation into the standard medical model, (2) partial integration, and (3) team care.

Selective Integration

Many observers, physicians in particular, accept that there can be (indeed should be) integration of *selected* aspects of complementary/alternative care into the mainstream. This will not be a modality in its entirety, but only those aspects that are supported by scientific and clinical evidence. This is fostered by the calls for a single set of standards for all health care and growing interest among complementary/alternative practitioners in "gold standard" clinical trials and evidence-based medicine, as discussed in Chapter 2.[58] It will, however, be a long time before there is unassailable evidence to dampen countless physician concerns over the "risks of embracing alternative medicine," particularly in relation to the quality of care, of products, and of research.[59]

Surveys generally show that physicians believe the current medical mind-set must remain predominant. A British report about integration, based on the views of directors of public health and representatives of general practitioner National Health Service fundholding consortiums, found the following five criteria were most frequently thought to be necessary for integration:

1. Effectiveness
2. Positive outcome studies
3. Cost-effectiveness
4. Recognized accreditation procedures and professional standards
5. Availability of qualified practitioners[60]

Much less importance was attached to meeting patient preferences, demands, or expectations.

Such survey information reminds us that, as already indicated, any selective integration makes many complementary/alternative practitioners uncomfortable because of the potential for it to become a steam-roller that will amount to a "take-over" by conventional medicine; this, it is said, will then dilute or remove the holistic approaches of most complementary/alternative modalities.

Partial Integration

This approach to integration follows the existing situations of mainstream "limited" professions such as dentistry, podiatry, optometry, psychology, speech therapy, and audiology. These professions are characterized by their practitioners being licensed to see patients without medical referral, albeit with their practices limited in two ways: to the parts of the human body they treat, and to a restricted range of techniques, instruments or therapies. Although various complementary/alternative medicine modalities have moved or are seemingly moving in this direction (e.g., chiropractic),[61] it must be asked whether limited medical professions actually serve integration, or merely entrench separate groups and encourage further specialization. Already within many complementary/alternative modalities subspecialization exists. Herbal medicine, for example, has its ardent proponents of what is called phytotherapy, which, in leading to selective integration of individual herbs or constituents into conventional medicine, moves herbal usage away from traditional herbalism.[62]

Team Care

We give particular attention to this third model for integration in Chapter 7 (team care). In effect, ideal team care between mainstream and complementary/alternative care would refine the partial integration model, in so far as practitioners would collaborate to bring together different practices to suit the individual needs of a patient. Team care is not easy, at least within hospital settings, largely because of concerns over lack of demonstrably consistent standards within complementary/alternative medicine,[63] and because treatment is often seen more as applying a regimen rather than as a social process. [64]

General Comments

Clearly, the extent to which integration will or will not occur within the first decade of the twenty-first century is an open issue as is also underscored in other sections of this book. A host of factors are at play as we have made clear. In summary we might stress (1) the general spirit of reform in health care among the general public, all practitioners, and governments, (2) whether or not physicians (and other health care professionals) become better informed and educated in complementary/alternative care (perhaps through changes in medical education), and (3) the results of new research (and research initiatives underway) on efficacy.

We conclude this section with emphasis on the subtle influences of cultural factors that can affect integration. We have noted already that the cultural characteristics of the U.S. provide an interesting comparison with Canada. Although cultural differences are not dramatic, subtle differences can be significant. In unending debates about the Canadian identity, the Canadian health care system is an important issue. There is general agreement that a scaffolding of legislation—the Canadian Charter of Rights and Freedoms, the Canada Health Act, and the Multiculturalism Act—creates distinctive features to the country's culture and health care system, certainly compared to the United States. Aside from five oft-quoted values or principles of the Canada Health Act (public administration, comprehensiveness, universality, portability, and accessibility), the scaffolding serves as a constant reminder of how the public values equality and justice irrespective of age, gender, and ethnicity. We suggest that together with what Canadians like to believe is part of Canadian culture—a sense of compromise—such values temporize and moderate both lay and professional opposition to complementary/alternative medicine and extreme anti-medicine views and hence may facilitate integration. Temporizing has a pedigree of sorts in the relatively muted Canadian opposition to alternative practices in the past. Canadian physicians in general, from c.1850-c.1940, were seemingly less vigorous in their opposition to various forms of alternative medicine, indeed almost ambivalent, compared with their U.S. counterparts.

NOTES

1. C. Webster, *The National Health Service,* Oxford: Oxford University Press, 1998, p. 69.

2. For an indication of widespread interest in the issues the House of Commons Standing Committee on Health Minutes, 1997-1998.

3. Definition of values adapted from various authors, especially W. K. Frankena, *Ethics,* Englewood Cliffs, NJ: Prentice-Hall, 1963.

4. Compare, D. W. Brock and N. Daniels, "Ethical Foundations of the Clinton Administration's Proposed Health Care System," *JAMA,* 1994; 271, 1189-1196; N. Daniels, "The Articulation of Values and Principles Involved in Health Care Reform," *Journal of Medicine and Philosophy,* 1994; 19, 425-433.

5. This is a common concern, but this quotation from Canadian AIDS Society, see House of Commons Standing Committee on Health Minutes, February 17, 1998, p. 6.

6. News release: <http://www.cpso.on.ca/newsrelease/NR-krop99.htm> (accessed September 2001).

7. We perhaps should add here that some commentators, at least, consider that present-day affluence contributes to the popularity of complementary/alternative care. For example, E. Ernst, letter to the editor, *Annals of Internal Medicine,* 1999; 131, 230.

8. See S. M. Weitzman, "Insurance Coverage for Complementary and Alternative Medicine: Access, Challenges and Policy," in J. M. Humber and R. F. Almeder, *Alternative Medicine and Ethics* Totowa, NJ: Humana Press, 1998, pp. 127-161. Many frustrations exist in the United States on differing attitudes among insurance companies and HMOs. As an example, "Soul Care," *Hospitals and Health Networks* 1999 (June 20) notes that a Denver HMO has made spiritual counseling a covered benefit. For failure of insurance companies to cover dietary supplements also marketed as pharmaceuticals, G. Kolata, "Drug or Food? Patients Stumble into Gray Area," *The New York Times,* February 9, 1999, p. D6. Differences of opinion exist in Canada and Britain over coverage under national insurance schemes, but users generally believe that it is important.

9. For Canada, CTV/Angus Reid poll, August 1997 ("Use of Alternative Medicine and Practices," <http://www.angusreid.com>, Web site accessed January 1998, survey no longer available), indicating that 70 percent of Canadians agreed ("strongly," 33 percent; "somewhat," 37 percent) with the statement that "our provincial health care plans should pay for alternative medicines and practices the same way that they pay for treatments and medicines prescribed by doctors." For U.S. survey by Interactive Solutions sponsored by Landmark Healthcare, Inc., Business Wire Health Wire, January 27, 1998.

10. This point was frequently made throughout House of Commons Standing Committee on Health Minutes, 1997-1998.

11. For example, P. Manga, "Defending the Manga Report on the Chiropractic Management of Low-Back Pain," *Canadian Medical Association Journal,* 1994; 151, 1250-1251. More recent controversies surround results published by: T. S. Carey, J. Garrett, A. Jackman, C. McLaughlin, J. Fryer, and D. R. Smucker, "The Outcomes and Costs of Care for Acute Low Back Pain Among Patients Seen by Primary Care Practitioners, Chiropractors, and Orthopedic Surgeons," *New England Journal of Medicine,* 1995; 333, 913-917; and D. C. Cherkin, R. A. Deyo, M. Battié, J. Street, and W. Barlow, "A Comparison of Physical Therapy, Chiropractic Manipulation, and Provision of an Educational Booklet for the Treatment of Patients with Low Back Pain," *New England Journal of Medicine,* 1998; 339, 1021-1029. The latter has been widely quoted along the lines that it has contributed to increasing doubts whether chiropractic is helpful for acute uncomplicated low back pain in a clinically relevant way. (For example, E. Ernst, "Complementary Medicine: Too Good to Be True?" *Journal of the Royal Society of Medicine,* 1999; 92, 1-2.) As anticipated, chiropractic practitioners have criticized the study on various grounds. For instance, a limited patient pool, delay in treatment, limitation of chiropractic to one procedure.

For delay in treatment issue: T. J. Kaptchuk and D. M. Eisenberg, "Chiropractic Origins, Controversies and Contributions," *Archives Internal Medicine,* 1998; 158, 2215-2224.

12. On methodology: A. R. White, "Economic Evaluation of Homeopathy," in E. Ernst and E. G. Hahn, eds., *Homeopathy: A Critical Appraisal,* Oxford: Butterworth-Heinemann, 1998, pp. 211-220; also, A. R. White, "Do Complementary Therapies Offer Value for Money?" in E. Ernst, ed., *Complementary Medicine: An Objective Appraisal,* Oxford: Butterworth-Heinemann, 1996, pp. 89-105 for quote. Some tentative provisos are offered. E. Ernst, "The Ethics of Complementary Medicine," *Journal of Medical Ethics,* 1996; 22, 197-198.

13. These opinions expressed in testimony before the House of Commons Standing Committee on Health Minutes, February 17, 1998, p. 28.

14. Health Canada has a guideline (2000) allowing importation of a three-month supply for personal use.

15. House of Commons Standing Committee on Health Minutes, February 17, 1998, p. 18. The attitudes of physicians to fibromyalgia are raised in a number of studies, e.g., O. Hellström, J. Burlington, G. Karlsson, P. Lindqvist, and B. Mattson, "Doctors Attitudes to Fibromyalgia: A Phenomenological Study," *Scandinavian Journal of Social Medicine,* 1998, 26(3), 232-237.

16. Angus Reid Poll. (Only 6 percent of the 42 percent of users indicated that they did not trust modern medicine and practices).

17. T. Pergola and S. Gailing, "The Role of Science in the Dietary Supplement Arena," *Natural Sensibility* [Hartman Group], 1999, newsletter 7 (February).

18. C. Vincent and A. Furnham, *Complementary Medicine: A Research Perspective,* Chichester: Wiley and Sons, 1997, pp. 105-108.

19. D. Irvine, "The Performance of Doctors. I: Professionalism and Self-Regulation in a Changing World," *BMJ,* 1997; 314, 1540-1542; and "II: Maintaining Good Practice. Protecting Patients from Poor Practice," *BMJ,* 1997; 314, 1613-1615.

20. J. Lazarou, B. H. Pomeranz, and P. N. Conrey, "Incidence of Adverse Drug Reactions in Hospitalized Patients," *JAMA,* 1998; 279, 1200-1205.

21. House of Commons Standing Committee on Health Minutes, March 10, 1998, pp. 30-31.

22. The minutes of the House of Commons Standing Committee on Health (1997-1998) reveal this view on many occasions. For reference to "state of rot," minutes March 12, 1998, p. 14. For concerns over Health Protection Branch from another perspective, J. Lexchin, "Secrecy and the Health Protection Branch," *Canadian Medical Association Journal,* 1998; 159, 481-483.

23. H. T. Stelfox, G. Chua, K. O'Rourke, and A. S. Detsky, "Conflict of Interest in the Debate Over Calcium-Channel Antagonists," *New England Journal of Medicine,* 1998; 338, 101-106.

24. House of Commons Standing Committee on Health Minutes, February 5, 1998, p. 28.

25. See conference report, J. Stephenson, "Medical Journals Turn Gaze Inward to Examine Process of Peer Review," *JAMA,* 1997; 278, 1389-1391. For other background: J. Barnes, N.C. Abbot, E.F. Harkness, and E. Ernst, "Articles on Complementary Medicine in the Mainstream Medical Literature," *Archives Internal Medicine,* 1999; 159, 1721-1725.

26. For overview, "Interpretation" in W.T. Reich, ed., *Encyclopedia of Bioethics*, New York: Simon and Schuster Macmillan, 1995, Volume 3, pp. 1283-1288.

27. S. Bosely, "Is Nanny Getting Her Vitamins in a Twist?" *Guardian Weekly*, August 2, 1998, p. 11. The debate also centered on the assessment of "scientific evidence," for example, J. Collier, "Vitamin B-6: Food or Medicine?" *BMJ*, 1998; 317, 92-93 and subsequent correspondence on article, BMJ, 1999; 318, 463-464.

28. H. Boon, "Canadian Naturopathic Practitioners: Holistic and Scientific World Views," *Social Science and Medicine*, 1998; 46, 1213-1225. It is relevant to add that those who practice acupuncture may rationalize their work on the basis of traditional Chinese theory or on Western science of physiology and biochemistry. Also, for subgroups, P. Tovey and J. Adams, "Thinking Sociologically about Complementary Medicine," *Complementary Therapies in Medicine*, 1999; 7, 113-115; and "Worlds of Difference: Towards a Grassroots Focus for the Study of Complementary Medicine in Primary Care," in T. Tovey, ed., *Contemporary Primary Care: The Challenge of Change 2000*, Buckingham: Open University Press, 1999.

29. On different attitudes to two cultures, E. Ernst *(Complementary Therapies in Medicine*, 1997; 5, 184) says they are so obvious they do not need comment. Others believe they are overstated.

30. For background, C. E. Rosenberg, "Pathologies of Progress: The Idea of Civilisation at Risk," *Bulletin of the History of Medicine*, 1998; 72, 714-730.

31. As part of our emphasis on critical appraisal, we believe that arguments supporting a wide range of symptoms (e.g., headaches, runny nose, joint pains, irritated eyes) being due to toxins in the body need careful examination. Do the views reflect traditional concepts or clinical/scientific evidence?

32. Considered in a review by T. J. Kaptchuck and D. M. Eisenberg, "The Persuasive Appeal of Alternative Medicine," *Annals of Internal Medicine*, 1998; 129, 1061-1070.

33. P. H. Ray first published observations on "The Emerging Culture" in 1997; for full discussion of a thesis that has attracted much discussion, P. H. Ray and S. R. Anderson, *The Cultural Creatives: How 50 Million People are Changing the World*, New York: Harmony Books, 2001.

34. For example, M. Baum, "What Is Holism? The View of a Well-Known Critic of Alternative Medicine," *Complementary Therapies in Medicine*, 1998; 6, 42-44.

35. Of interest among software programs for homeopathy is one with the imprimatur of George Vithoulkas, an internationally-known authority within the field (RADAR: <www.wholehealthnow.com> accessed September 2001).

36. J. Hoey, "The Arrogance of Science and the Pitfalls of Hope," *Canadian Medical Association Journal*, 1998; 159, 803-804, wrote: "When passion edges into zeal and frustration becomes arrogance, scientists lose credibility and risk depriving us of their considerable and unique understanding of the intricacies of biology and the nuances of meaningful research."

37. J. S. Goodwin and M. R. Tangum, "Battling Quackery. Attitudes About Micronutrient Supplements in American Academic Medicine," *Archives Internal Medicine*, 1998; 158, 2187-2191. Statements such as "there are people who simply believe supplements generally aren't useful and if you eat a well-balanced diet there is no need to take additional vitamins and minerals" also reveal ideological tensions. (House of Commons Standing Committee on Health Minutes, March 24, 1998, p. 46.)

38. For discussion on heresy: P. R. Wolpe, "The Dynamics of Heresy in a Profession," *Social Science and Medicine,* 1994; 39, 1133-1148.

39. For comments on prudence, S-T. Teo, S. Torng, and J. K. Crellin, "Health Food Stores: Pathways to Alternative Medicine," in *Proceedings of VIII International Conference on Traditional Medicine and Folklore, St. John's 1994,* St. John's: Faculty of Medicine, Memorial University, Volume 2, pp. 91-98.

40. Compare C. Vincent and A. Furnham, *Complementary Medicine: A Research Perspective,* Chichester: Wiley and Sons, 1997, p. 77.

41. See, for example, C. Lawrence and G. Weisz, *Greater Than the Parts: Holism in Biomedicine, 1920-1950,* New York: Oxford University Press, 1998.

42. For typical discussion, T. Brewin, "Use of the Word 'Scientific,'" *Lancet,* 2000; 355, 586; and V.S. Rambihar, "Science, Evidence, and the Use of the Word Scientific," *Lancet,* 2000; 355, 1730.

43. Vincent and Furnham, *Complementary Medicine,* p. 110.

44. For review, albeit without current emphasis on holism: R. C. Kelvinson, "Colonic Hydrotherapy: A Review of the Available Literature," *Complementary Therapies in Medicine,* 1995; 3 (April), 88-92.

45. Published goals of the British Holistic Medical Association.

46. Baum, "What Is Holism?"

47. House of Commons Standing Committee on Health Minutes, March 25, 1998, p. 17, comments from the Traditional Healers Committee, Opasquick Cree Nation, Canada.

48. J. Stone and J. Matthews, *Complementary Medicine and the Law,* Oxford: Oxford University Press, 1996, p. 208. See also M. Saks, "Alternative Therapies: Are They Holistic?" *Complementary Therapies in Nursing and Midwifery,* 1997; 3, 4-8.

49. Following the withdrawal of Russian economic support Cuba undertook a "green revolution" toward herbal medicine. Although it is widely believed that China and Japan have greater integration of conventional and complementary/alternative medicine than in the West, some consider the integration is not so complete as imagined. Compare, for instance, M. Matsumato, K. Inoue, and E. Kajii, "Integrating Traditional Medicine in Japan: The Case of Kampo Medicines," *Complementary Therapies in Medicine,* 1999; 7, 254-255. In China, questions arise whether traditional medicine has been adapted to allow it to run as a parallel system to Western medicine, see V. Scheid, "The Globalisation of Chinese Medicine," *Supplement to Lancet 2000,* 1999 (December), Siv 10.

50. For example, C. A. Schroeder and J. Likkel, "Integrative Health Care: The Revolution Is Upon Us," *Public Health Nursing,* 1999; 16, 233-234. In contrast to statements such as "As long as there remain chiropractors who maintain a profoundly anti-scientific approach to health-care, there is little chance of ever bridging the rift between the two professions, no matter how devoutly the majority of practitioners on both sides might wish it." ("Who Will Bridge the Gap Between Chiropractors and Doctors?" *The Medical Post,* 2000; 36 [February 8], 13).

51. A recent review from the United States stated that integration can range from 9 percent for homeopathy to 19 percent for chiropractic (practices which receive vigorous challenges from medicine) and massage therapy not seen as a threat to conventional medicine. J. A. Astin, A. Marie, K. R. Pelletier, E. Hansen, and W. L. Haskell, "A Review of the Incorporation of Complementary and Alternative Medicine by Mainstream Physicians," *Archives of Internal Medicine,* 1998; 158, 2303-

2310. For other information on massage, M. J. Verhoef and S. A. Page, in "Physicians' Perspectives on Massage Therapy," *Canadian Family Physician*, 1998; 44, 1018-1024, find that although Alberta physicians have little knowledge of massage they generally hold positive opinions of it. It should be added that nursing has been far more accommodating to many aspects (especially mind-body) of complementary/alternative medicine. Compare, for example, textbooks such as M. Snyder and R. Lindquist, *Complementary/Alternative Therapies in Nursing*, New York: Springer, 1998.

52. W. B. Jonas, "Alternative Medicine—Learning from the Past, Examining the Present, Advancing to the Future," *JAMA*, 1998, 280, 1616-1618. Discussions on integration extend to changes within conventional medicine, both micro and macro levels, e.g., R. Snyderman and V. Y. Seito, *Integrating Health Care Delivery Systems*, Durham: Duke University Medical Center and Health Systems, 1998. Earlier references to attract much interest include J. W. LaValley and M. J. Verhoef, "Integrating Complementary Medicine into Conventional Practice," *Canadian Medical Association Journal*, 1995; 153, 45-49. They make the interesting distinction: complementary medicine is offered solely by physicians; and complementary health care by any practitioner.

53. H. Brody, J. M. Rygwelski, and M. D. Fetters, "Ethics at the Interface of Conventional and Complementary Medicine," in W. B. Jonas and J. S. Levin, eds., *Essentials of Complementary and Alternative Medicine*, Philadelphia: Lippincott Williams and Wilkins, 1999, pp. 46-56.

54. Compare a view published by the Foundation for Integrated Medicine: *Integrated Health Care: A Way Forward for the Next Five Years, A Discussion Document*, 1997, p. 4.

55. For example, D. M. Eisenberg, R. B. Davis, S. L. Ettner, S. Appel, S. Wilkey, M. V. Rompey, and R. C. Kessler, "Trends in Alternative Medicine Use in the United States, 1990-1997. Results of a Follow-Up National Survey," *JAMA*, 1998; 280, 1569-1575.

56. Some of these ideas echo the assessments of certain physicians. See S. R. Kaufman, *The Healer's Tale: Transforming Medicine and Culture*, Madison: University of Wisconsin Press, 1993, various pages. For others who note fragmentation in general, A. Best and C. Herbert, "Two Solitudes of Complementary and Conventional Medicine: Where Are We Going?" *Canadian Family Physician*, 1998; 44, 953-955.

57. A variety of developments promoting integrative programs are worthy of close attention to assess their influence, such as The University of Arizona Program in Integrative Medicine that focuses on training physicians in integrative medicine.

58. I. Chalmers, "Evidence of the Effects of Health Care: A Plea for a Single Standard Across 'Orthodox' and 'Complementary' Medicine," *Complementary Therapies in Medicine*, 1998; 6, 211-213. Aside from emphasizing the role of the Cochrane collaboration the writer added that "the most important resource required to promote the concept of integrated health care is likely to be humility among those whose practices will be put to the test, within both orthodox and complementary medicine." Compare, also, J. E. Dalen, "'Conventional' and 'Unconventional' Medicine: Can They Be Integrated?" *Archives of Internal Medicine*, 1998; 158, 2179-2181.

59. W. B. Jonas, "Safety in Complementary Medicine" in E. Ernst, ed., *Complementary Medicine: An Objective Appraisal,* Oxford: Butterworth-Heinemann, 1996, pp. 126-149.

60. E. Ernst, N. C. Armstrong, A. R. White, and M. H. Pittler, "Research Is Needed to Determine How to Integrate Complementary Medicine into the NHS," *BMJ,* 1998; 317, 1654. Another study indicates that "general practice is responding to complementary medicine by trying out the more 'respectable' therapies (in terms of scientific method and evidence.") A. M. Wearn and S. M. Greenfield, "Access to Complementary Medicine in General Practice: Survey in One UK Health Authority," *Journal of the Royal Society of Medicine,* 1998; 91, 465-470.

61. W. I. Wardwell, "Chiropractic in the Twenty-First Century," in D. Peterson and G. Wiese, eds., *Chiropractic: An Illustrated History,* St. Louis: Mosby, 1995, pp. 489-495 (p. 491).

62. As an example of focusing on constituents, and trends away from traditional herbal medicine, J. D. Phillipson in "Radioligand-Receptor Binding Assays in the Search for Bioactive Principles from Plants," *Journal of Pharmacy and Pharmacology,* 1999, 51, 493-503, indicates new assay methods to identify plant constituents with specific actions on cell receptors.

63. This is pointed out in various places, e.g., *Integrated Healthcare: A Way Forward for the Next Five Years,* London: The Foundation for Integrated Medicine, 1998.

64. A. Mitchell and M. Cormack, *The Therapeutic Relationship in Complementary Health Care,* Edinburgh: Churchill Livingstone, 1998.

Chapter 4

Standards of Care:
A Need for Critical Skills

STANDARDS OF CARE, THE COURTS,
AND COMPLEMENTARY/ALTERNATIVE MEDICINE

Although standards are another aspect of calls for change, we treat them separately as more a matter of professionalism. In many ways this book could be titled "standards of care," although it might then be misconstrued as dealing only with the technical aspects of complementary/alternative medicine. Standards must imply that appropriate procedures are not only implemented, but also applied sensitively and ethically. One reason for focusing on "standards" (and a lack of them) is that they increasingly became a public issue in the 1980s and 1990s through malpractice suits, the growing costs of health care services, and a new emphasis on accountability of practitioners.

Courts have increasingly been involved in examining the standards of medical practice. In the United States, Canada, and Britain it has been established that acceptable standards of care for conventional medicine are those followed by a responsible body of medical opinion. Moreover, a general practitioner, for instance, is held to the standards of general practice, not of specialist care.[1] Putting this another way, a "reasonable" standard for physicians is the "duty to conduct their practice in accordance with the conduct of a prudent and diligent doctor in the same circumstances."[2] Of course, terms such as reasonable, diligent, and prudent can be nuanced in various ways. Prudent, for instance, can imply conservative practices and the avoidance of relatively untested approaches, whereas others may see the same untested approaches as being in the best interests of a patient. Yet whatever courtroom interpretations might be made over whether standards have been violated—and disagreements between medical "experts" are no-

torious—diligence and prudence always underpin a practitioner's responsibility to evaluate carefully his or her level of care.

With regard to complementary/alternative medicine, the courts will not generally apply the standards of care established for the conventional medical profession. Instead the specific standards established for each modality would be accepted.[3] However, this prompts the question: Are appropriate practice standards established in all areas of complementary/alternative care? Unfortunately, the answer is "No."[4] Even where they exist, problems may still arise. For instance, although the licenses of chiropractors may limit the scope of practice to the spine, many of them offer a wide variety of other treatments.[5] Chiropractors have long been divided into "straights" and "mixers," the latter commonly embracing many modalities beyond traditional spinal manipulation. Acupuncturists may use "modern" rather than traditional acupuncture. Not surprisingly, debates, which need resolution, exist on "What is an acupuncturist?" "What is a naturopath?"[6] and "When is an aromatherapist not an aromatherapist?"[7]

Even greater uncertainties about standards exist where there is no statutory licensing. Indeed, the absence of this even makes such terms as "professional standards" problematic, since courts accept licensing as a criterion of being a "professional." Moreover, the individuality of many practitioners can make it difficult to find agreement over practice standards as when, for example, a therapist claims roles for intuition or spiritual forces when making a diagnosis. In the absence of licensing, courts have applied the standards of conventional medicine, which may well mean verdicts of practicing medicine without a license.[8]

Having raised questions about standards of complementary/alternative medicine, it must be said that this has not yet become a public matter largely because malpractice suits against its practitioners have not become a major issue. A 1998 report stated that "alternative medicine accounts for approximately 5 percent of the total medical malpractice market in the U.S."[9] However, the general concern with standards and the growing public emphasis on accountability must alert all practitioners to ensure standards of "prudent and diligent practice." A law textbook (1998) indicates that the present situation of relatively little litigation over complementary medicine in any jurisdiction is likely to change and that consideration needs to be given to standards of formulation, manufacture, promotion and prescribing. The authors note that "any health practitioner, whether certified in

any manner or not, who makes use of an unregistered product in the course of his/her treatment, and who has assumed full responsibility for the patient and his therapy, is likely to be held answerable for any ill consequences which this treatment may have."[10] At the same time, a physician may face legal proceedings if he or she refers a patient to an inadequately qualified practitioner who provides negligent care.[11] Standards, too, can be undone by errors. Should the patient be told of these errors whether they are detrimental or not? The answer is generally yes, on the moral grounds of respecting the patient and telling the truth. Moreover, if information is withheld and an impression of a cover-up is discovered by the patient, the scene may be set for malpractice and/or disciplinary hearings.

We should mention here an obvious consideration, that all health care providers are subject to laws of general application, from criminal matters to consumer protection. Unfortunately for patients, in most jurisdictions, any action against a practitioner is one of civil liability, which is an expensive process. Indeed, two Canadian lawyers have written (1999) that the "potential lack of compensation for the victims of incompetent or unethical practice by those who offer alternative therapies seems to make a very strong case for regulation of health care providers."[12]

Further matters about standards are raised, directly and indirectly, in various places in this volume. Next, however, we look particularly at safety and related issues; as has been said, "critical ethical concerns regarding safety and efficacy" need careful consideration.[13]

SAFETY AND STANDARDS

Introduction

Because discussions on safety most commonly focus on herbs and dietary supplements, a sense exists that safety is concerned only with toxic constituents or incompatibilities with prescription products. However, a variety of issues must be evaluated whenever safety risks are considered. For example:

1. The accuracy of the diagnosis
2. The context in which a product is used, such as in self-care or under the care of a professional who has appropriate skills in diagnosis and therapeutics

3. The potential treatment benefits relative to risks
4. The marketing, advertising, or advice and whether it leads to inappropriate treatment
5. The appropriateness of a treatment for different groups of patients, such as children or the elderly
6. A practitioner's ability to recognize subjective judgements about a treatment (for instance, apparent toxic effects from herbal products have been interpreted by patients as symptoms of the condition that they are treating)
7. The state of health of a subject and what are appropriate interventions, bearing in mind possible interactions between multiple treatments[14]

Diagnosis

Among the many safety considerations misdiagnosis can be as critical as unsafe treatments. Moreover, diagnosis is a special issue within complementary/alternative medicine, especially for non-MD practitioners, since making a diagnosis is commonly viewed as being at the heart of whether one is "practicing medicine" or not. In many jurisdictions in the United States and Canada, the specific act of making a diagnosis opens up possible charges of practicing medicine without a license. We notice later (under Oaths and Codes in Chapter 6) that differences of opinion exist over whether complementary/alternative practitioners should make diagnoses.

A complicating issue is that the term "diagnosis" can have different meanings, at least different diagnostic classifications (e.g., mainstream, homeopathic, and traditional Chinese medicine.) In 1976, a nonphysician homeopath in California successfully defended a charge of practicing medicine without a license on the grounds that homeopathy, because of its different theory and therapy, is not mainstream medicine in which diagnosis depends on correlating signs and symptoms with specific pathology.[15] Many complementary/alternative practitioners clearly do not recognize conventional diagnoses ("I am not talking about a diagnosis because I am only dealing with energy"). It is argued, too, that since much complementary/alternative health care only assists the body to heal itself, specific diagnoses are not essential.

Those complementary/alternative practitioners who work within the framework of conventional physiological concepts (e.g., herbalists who base their practice on active constituents) may deliberately sidestep the language of diagnosis to avoid charges of practicing medicine. They say they take "health," rather than "medical," histories in ways that help patients educate themselves about their condition; in other words they do little more than many patients have learned or are learning to do for themselves. Furthermore, some say many aspects of a physical examination, such as a speculum inspection of the vagina and cervix, are no different from what some women—influenced by the Women's Health Movement of recent decades—use in self-care. Another example is measuring blood pressure, which is seen as "the same as patients taking their own blood pressure in any store."[16]

Concern is sometimes expressed over the ready way some mainstream practitioners, who practice complementary/alternative medicine, shift from one diagnostic classification scheme to another. Also, those who practice, for instance, acupuncture (especially physicians) often ignore Chinese theory and approaches to diagnosis. Although practitioners (and many patients) are comfortable with such an empirical approach ("it works"), this may overlook evidence that, at times, theoretical-based approaches in complementary/alternative medicine have offered benefits to patients when conventional treatments have failed. Clearly a good understanding of *all* approaches to diagnostic classifications can add to quality care. To this we add the importance of recognizing relevant social factors; for instance, why some diseases seem to be fashionable at times (e.g., hypoglycemia comes and goes) and why certain diagnoses are more prevalent in certain countries than others.

Some commentators say that a broad understanding of diagnostic classifications is particularly significant for complementary/alternative practitioners who must at least have a good understanding of mainstream approaches. Licensed physicians, who are upset over what they see to be the minimal training in diagnosis among complementary/alternative students, constantly stress that, even after their own long years of training, making a diagnosis can be elusive. This leads many, albeit without consideration of different approaches to diagnosis, to call for licensing of all complementary/alternative practitioners so as to ensure they have sufficient skills to recognize the limits of help they can give to patients and when to refer to conventional medicine. Recognizing limits is a particular responsibility for students of complementary/alternative medicine (indeed for all wise health care students), who often feel that their education provides an insufficient "comfort level" to make the transition from student to solo practitioner.

We complete these notes with comments by M. Tierra, a prominent U.S. writer on herbs, who seemingly tries to build bridges. He recognizes that clinical judgement or intuition in diagnosis (see Oaths and Codes, in Chapter 6) is often referred to by complementary/alternative practitioners ("practices such as kinesiology, radionics, and iridology, focus more on the intuitive side of diagnosis"). However, in referring to these and other modalities, he is concerned with those practitioners whose methodological approach does not begin with data: "My approach is to evaluate all that is possible of the known and continue to extend gradually to the more intuitive level of knowing."[17]

Herbs/Natural Health Products

That herbal safety dominates discussions on safety of complementary/alternative medicine is not inappropriate in so far as herbs are recommended and administered not only by herbalists, but also by acupuncturists, chiropractors, homeopaths, naturopaths, and other practitioners, as well as being used by countless individuals as part of their self-care. Further, there is the issue—confusing to many laypeople—that herbs and their products are sold either as medicines, ingredients in functional foods, dietary supplements, and so on. Mislabeled and inferior quality, or badly adulterated products also add concerns. A particular worry is whether or not the same safety considerations should apply to the great variety of dietary supplements that include homeopathic preparations, vitamins, minerals, enzymes, co-enzymes, co-factors, herbs or botanicals, animal source substances, and a variety of molecules extracted from natural substances such as amino acids, polysaccharides, peptides, naturally occurring hormones and precursors as well as naturally occurring molecules synthesized by chemical or biological means.[18]

Although supporters of complementary/alternative medicine often argue that, in many jurisdictions, existing government controls of herbs/dietary supplements are overly protective, others consider that legislation should be strengthened, or implemented more consistently, in order to protect the public. Finding the right balance between these two views—especially when there is vigorous conflict over the safety of particular products—is difficult. A professional responsibility may well exist to become involved in public education about the complexity of such issues. For instance, a need surely existed during the already mentioned 1998 British controversy over the safety of large doses of vitamin B_6. In contrast, relatively little disagreement arises over the dangers of "traditional" Chinese medicines adulterated with steroids and heavy metals.[19]

Some observers take the view that the evaluation and standardization of pharmaceuticals—with its rigorous approach to determining toxicities at particular dose levels over short- and long-term usage—should be, despite the high costs, the model for complementary/alternative products. However, others consider that such an exhaustive approach is unnecessary and that the relatively few reported side effects from natural health products are not placed in the context of the strikingly high incidence of prescription drug side effects. Although this is correct, it is questionable to use the information to rebut statements that there cannot be different standards of safety (and efficacy) between complementary/alternative and conventional medicine.[20] After all, concerns of widespread underreporting of side effects of herbs and of interactions or incompatabilities with prescription drugs must be examined carefully.[21] By 2000, these had become a conspicuous issue through reports of a wide range of examples such as the apparently safe St. John's wort interacting with other antidepressants, antibiotics, anticoagulants, oral contraceptives, and immunosuppressives.[22]

A further safety concern of the late 1990s—a by-product of uncontrolled marketing and promotion—was the accuracy of information provided to customers visiting health food stores.[23] This goes beyond false information to such subtle, open-ended questions as, "Can you be sure that you are taking enough zinc, or vitamin E?" The latter, in the absence of clear answers, creates uncertainty and may encourage both unnecessary usage and large doses. Lastly, we note that, despite the general acceptance (legally and popularly) of the term dietary supplement, complementary/alternative practitioners need to ask if the term is really justified for herbs that have long histories as medicinals. Do such terms as "traditional medicines" suggest there should be a prudent approach to safety?

Other Safety Issues, Including Inappropriate Personal Relationships

Although herbs/dietary supplements attract most attention, concerns exist about the safety of almost all other modalities. For instance, chiropractic's public image suffered in 1998 when *Maclean's,*

Canada's weekly news magazine, banner headlined a story of a rare complication of a ruptured vertebral artery in a twenty-year-old woman: "Lethal treatment. The death of a patient puts chiropractic on trial."[24] Fear mongering aside, the medical literature records many safety problems with chiropractic (although without comparable comparisons with conventional medical outcomes). What becomes clear is the ethical need for specific informed consent (see related discussion in Chapter 7) prior to particular treatments such as cervical manipulation with thrust techniques that arouse particular concerns.[25] Worries also exist over invasive practices (e.g., trauma and infection as a result of acupuncture).

Even noninvasive aromatherapy and noninvasive mind-body therapies (e.g., meditation, yoga, and focusing) raise concerns.[26] In fact, mind-body approaches are generally overlooked for potential safety problems, as is the view that intercessionary prayer might have adverse effects.[27] Also commonly ignored are potential difficult-to-resolve psychological problems whenever patients (in treatment or counseling) are led to introspection or to having their hopes of recovery inappropriately raised. Often ignored, too, as a "safety" (rather than abuse) issue is personal (often sexual) relationships between practitioner and patient. Although practitioner-patient relationships are considered fully in Part II, we emphasize here that questionable situations generally violate the ethical principle that practitioners must do no harm to patients. A British MD-hypnotherapist's concern in 1996, made in the context of calls for greater regulation, is just one adverse report about unethical complementary/alternative practitioners; this is all the more worrisome, some argue, because of the widespread absence of licensing, of effective disciplinary procedures, and a sense of professionalism. After noting that although "physical harm is usually easily recognizable and corrected, [and] psychological harm can blight the remainder of a patient's life," the MD-hypnotherapist discussed a patient with "minor post-traumatic stress disorder as a result of advances made to her by a lay hypnotherapist against whom patients have made several allegations of sexual impropriety." Further, if prosecuted and convicted "there would be no means of preventing him from resuming practice."[28]

With regards to growing zero-tolerance over sexual abuse in Western societies, all practitioners must consider obtaining verbal consent every time a physical examination (especially of the breasts and genitals) is undertaken, even if consent for a general examination has already been obtained. Moreover, even where a high level of trust exists between practitioner and patient, such examinations probably should not be given without an attendant present unless written consent has been given.[29] Not all codes of ethics alert practitioners, as does the U.K. Institute of Complementary Medicine, in stating that patients are to be warned when "a specific treatment requires the removal of clothing where this is not immediately obvious." Aside from ensuring patient comfort, at issue is that, if practitioners touch patients in any way, when they have no authority or permission to do so, they lay themselves open to charges of battery.[30]

Safety of Homeopathic Medicines

We close our remarks on safety and standards with some comments on a question, Are homeopathic medicines safe? This helps to underscore the existence of many uncertainties in connection with safety. The view that homeopathic medicines are safe, because of their extreme dilutions, is widespread. Probably no nonhomeopath thinks otherwise. However, one survey (1998, unfortunately without any details) of over-the-counter complementary medicines used for arthritis notes that, at least six individuals (out of 1,020) reported adverse reactions to homeopathy.[31] This at least signals concern, as do a few studies on side effects of homeopathic remedies.[32] Allergic reactions from low potency preparations have been reported, as have potentially toxic concentrations of arsenic and cadmium albeit as reflections of careless manufacturing practices or deliberate adulteration.[33] Nevertheless, even critics recognize that side effects are rare, though long-term usage has received little careful study,[34] and that weak professional organizations in many jurisdictions, mean side effects are not being reported and compiled systematically. As well, additional issues are raised by experienced clinical homeopaths. For instance, (1) the failure to recognize an initial aggravation of symptoms on commencing treatment (a not uncommon phenomenon), and (2) problems from inappropriate homeopathic remedies being administered based on incorrect diagnoses or inappropriate dosages.

In the context of general concerns over homeopathy, Konstantin Keller, Director of the Federal Institute for Drugs and Medical Devises in Germany, highlighted a sharp contrast to North America:

> We [in Germany] think the strict control of the safety of homeopathic medicinal products is necessary because they may present

risks, and many homeopathic products on the German market
have been subject to pharmacovigilance action and have had to be
withdrawn from the market for safety reasons. We think homeopathic medicinal products should be included in pharmacovigilance systems as well. . . .[We] have had the experience now for
nearly 20 years that there is the need to protect public health in
this area.[35]

Many homeopaths outside Germany, sympathetic to more controls
than currently exist in their own jurisdictions, argue that only well-
educated and well-trained practitioners can (1) ascertain risks due to
aggravations from homeopathic medicines, (2) avoid prescribing inappropriate remedies and doses, and (3) decide when referral to a non-
homeopathic practitioner is in the best interests of a patient. The same
homeopaths also express concerns over most "high potency remedies" currently available over-the-counter in many pharmacies and
health food stores; opinions exist that such remedies should be fur-
nished on a prescription basis only.[36]

CRITICAL EVALUATION; HISTORICAL PEDIGREES

Another safety issue that needs critical appraisal is the often-repeated
view that complementary/alternative practices are safe (and/or effective) because they have been "around a long time," even back to the
"Bible." We elaborate on this topic here for a number of reasons. One
is that with our current lack of knowledge of constituents and of clinical studies—and that new information will not be forthcoming for
most herbs in the near future—a considerable reliance is being placed
on historical information. A second reason is that it is a matter of professional integrity to evaluate critically the historical record as much
as scientific data.

Widespread public belief indicates that usage, safety, and efficacy is
associated with, for example, American aboriginal, traditional Chinese, and herbal medicine in general. Many herbal "authorities" also
proclaim this view. Even from within the medical/pharmaceutical establishment, where a lot of suspicion exists over herbs, one can find
positive generalizations about historical information. For instance, a
dean of a pharmacy school acknowledged "the volumes of literature
and knowledge out there, accumulated through generations if not centuries of practice, that [could be] very reliable."[37] More explicit state-

ments exist: "the use of natural health products for sustained periods with long historical records shows that very largely they have a high safety margin and also a low risk."[38] The World Health Organization's *Guidelines for the Assessment of Herbal Medicines* states, "that if the product has been traditionally used without demonstrated harm no specific restrictive regulatory action should be undertaken unless new evidence demands a revised risk-benefit assessment."[39]

Another type of comment, in fact unsupportive of herbs, also encourages a mind-set that assumes herbal safety. This is the dismissal of the majority of "medicines and medical practices prior to the time of the twentieth century" as "inert."[40] Any reputation is said to be due to placebo action, which further pushes aside concerns over side effects.

One worrisome factor behind the frequency and authority of all such positive statements about historical safety is that they tend to close the mind to critical evaluations. In fact, while evaluations, based on established criteria, are one of the hallmarks of, say, medical science, there is little critical investigation of the historical record, a careful reading of which reveals many disagreements and uncertainties, especially about effectiveness.[41] Amid the search for positive statements, negative information is commonly overlooked, even though the latter may be based on extensive experience of practitioners at a time when herbs were the mainstay of conventional therapy. *Systematic* critical evaluation is necessary (see Box 4.1). Historians, in fact, rarely make pronouncements about herbal safety and effectiveness based on the historical record; at least, if they do it is with justifiable caution. After all, the entry on tobacco in the 1955 edition of Black's *Medical Dictionary* states that after "three centuries of experience [showing] comparative harmlessness of tobacco when used in moderation, equally violent diatribes are still being directed against smoking."[42] The change in attitudes toward the safety of smoking (inconsequence of new data) since 1955 has been, of course, dramatic. The tobacco and ill-health story in the twentieth century is also notable for the cigarette replacing the pipe, which serves as an indirect reminder that traditional health practices are never entirely constant. Indeed, herbal information currently recorded from traditional practitioners, even in remote places, often contains recent information, some appropriately described as "New Age." Contrarily, loss of traditional knowledge may include pertinent information on safety.

Despite the need to challenge the widespread confidence in the historical record, few critiques exist, though a useful "test of time"

BOX 4.1. Evaluating the Historical Record of Herbs

The text indicates that the historical record is commonly used superficially and uncritically. We add here some notes on some basic issues for systematic critical appraisal. Rarely considered are

1. tho divereity of listed uses of, say, an herbal medicine in the past;
2. that recommended uses were sometimes based on outdated theories and ultimately discarded during the heyday of usage of herbs in regular medicine; and
3. specific recommendation of dosages may reflect an appreciation of toxicity.

A critical evaluation of the historical record to determine ways in which an herb has been used in the past must consider the following:

1. Information from once widely used textbooks, which should span a long period of time (Those slavishly copied from other texts should be used cautiously. In other words, greatest attention should be given to books written by authors who themselves have critically evaluated the reputation of an herb or herbal medicine *at a time when the herb was in common use.*)
2. An assessment of stated uses for *each* preparation employed (powder, infusion, decoction, etc.) and for recommended dosages
3. A study, if possible, of records of usage by physicians, such as case notes, written when the herb was in general use (This contrasts with textbook information.)

An assessment of the historical reputation of an herb also needs to consider:

1. medical theories of the time (to what extent do recommended uses reflect theories rather than clinical observations?);
2. patients' expectations (was the herb, or a preparation of it, intended to provide relief of symptoms rather than a cure?); and
3. placebo response (was this recognized in the past as part of the reputation, and was it encouraged by the way an herb was recommended and administered?).

---

has been proposed[43] that emphasizes differences between past and present usages of herbs, and prompts questions about loss of traditional knowledge.[44] More specific challenges to the historical record can, unfortunately, be quite uncritical. One noteworthy example concerns the celebrated foxglove *(Digitalis purpurea).* In 1998, the President of the Canadian Medical Association agreed that a 1996 study—"a $40-

million or $50-million study, international, multi-centre trial"—
showed that "digitalis was not only dangerous, but it increased the
sudden deaths, the deaths out of hospital."[45] He indicated that there
had been no study in two hundred years whether it was safe or effective, and that digitalis would probably fall out of use within the next
five to ten years.[46]

These comments raise various instructive points, such that one won-
ders whether the physician's views were shaped by a professional bias
toward herbs. He disagreed with other commentators who stated "the
results of the trial should not lead most physicians to change their prescribing habits."[47] He also failed to notice that the new study was done
on digoxin, a glycoside from *Digitalis lanata,* not from the celebrated
foxglove, a different species, *Digitalis purpurea,* which, in fact, contains, as a main glycoside, digitoxin; and he did not appreciate that the
history of the use of foxglove as a heart medicine is hardly straightforward, and that its modern usage only dates from the early twentieth
century, not the late eighteenth century as commonly stated.

QUALITY AND STANDARDIZATION
OF PREPARATIONS

Considerations of the safety of natural health products go beyond
specific toxicities to worries over inferior quality. Not surprisingly,
with the increasing worldwide demand for herbs, intense commercial-
ization, sometimes short supplies, and failures to implement "good
manufacturing practices," the sale of incorrectly identified, adulterated or otherwise inferior quality products is widely reported. This,
long an issue in the medical literature, increasingly reaches the public
media, sometimes through government warnings (e.g., digitalis substituted for, or an adulterant of, plantain).[48] Clearly complemen-
tary/alternative practitioners must fear the possibility of large-scale
adverse publicity over some unfortunate mishap. After all, proponents of herbal medicine themselves can be heard to say that "a lack
of adequate regulation among herbal products leads to a confusing
mix of products, offering different dosages and dosing formats such
as capsules, teas and pills."[49]

At present, even where quality standards exist for herbs (sometimes voluntary ones implemented by companies, in the absence of
government regulations) there are problems.[50] Some relate to "im-

provement" in the quality of commercial herbal preparations in recent years due to "standardization." Indeed, much herbal promotion centers on the responsibility of using standardized preparations. Yet choosing from a range of preparations can be difficult, and challenges responsibilities when advising patients. For example, feverfew preparations for treating migraine, commercially available in 1999, included extracts, and extracts plus dried leaves in various-sized capsules that were mainly standardized to 0.2, 0.5, or 0.9 percent of "parthenolide."[51] A further issue is the relationship between the marker constituent and total pharmacological action. Clinical trials utilized parthenolide concentrations from 0.2 percent to 0.66 percent, but other constituents present may well have clinical value.[52]

In general, due to lack of detailed pharmacological and clinical studies, there is presently no guarantee that "marker" constituents contribute all or even part of the therapeutic potency of any herb. In other words, standardization is not a measure of potency. Phytochemists and herbalists point out, too, that methods of processing and preparing herbal preparations (e.g., freeze dried, air dried, water or hydroalcoholic extracts, juices, etc.) can lead to significantly different concentrations of constituents.[53] It is no surprise that many herbalists consider that selective extraction and standardization violates what they consider to be a central tenet of their practices, namely, the use of the whole plant. As one practitioner said recently, "the very core of our entire profession is based on one main defining principle, the use of whole plant constituents. I cannot reconcile the use of standardised herbal medicines. . . . I sincerely question whether 'standardising' our herbs, to conform to an allopathic framework, is the golden validation we need."[54] Herbalists, too, often place particular confidence in combination herbs for efficacy and safety, and argue that single herbs produce a higher percentage of adverse reactions. This is part of a widespread concern that the "modernization" of traditional herbal medicine is reducing it to the use of constituents and thereby losing traditional effects on the whole body.

The attention given to standardizing constituents—sometimes described as the European model of rational herbalism (or phytotherapy)—is characterized as the application of science to herbs and hence reductionist in nature. Tensions exist between this and other "schools" that base their teachings on, for instance, concepts of energy or nutritional profiles. These include popular views that "essences" of herbs are the natural "energies" that maintain or restore health by balancing or rebalancing the energy of the human body, and that "herbs are used for regulatory purposes [in the body], whereas drugs are used for killing a virus or bacteria."[55] Yet other practitioners see, as separate from or as part of the concept of energy balance, an essential role for plant "micronutrients." Herbs, according to some practitioners, are "very specialized foods for the cells of the body."[56] Such views of herbs and preparations that list concentrations of vitamins, minerals and fibers, can downplay concerns over toxicity.[57] Underlying the different perspectives just outlined are various ethical responsibilities, if only as an aspect of informed consent by making sure patients understand the particular rationale for their use of herbs.

EFFICACY, EFFECTIVENESS, AND PLACEBOS

A long-standing objective of regulatory bodies is to ensure safety, quality and efficacy of medicines. Many ask, however, whether efficacy should be part of the standards demanded for herbal products, or, for that matter, any complementary/alternative practice? If so, what standards of evidence of efficacy are required: clinical studies and their systematic review that, as already noted, are now the gold standard of evidence-based medicine (see Chapter 2), or historical data and testimonials? If efficacy is only marginal, should risk (safety) assessment be all the more rigorous? Alternatively, can "safe" products be evaluated for efficacy on the basis of relatively "soft" rather than "hard" evidence? After all, many argue that subjective satisfaction of consumers—such as feeling better, or "taking control" of their treatment—is a particularly important part of complementary/alternative care.[58] Unfortunately, difficulties in measuring satisfaction or "outcomes" can make this problematic. (It is noteworthy that the term "alterative" has become fashionable once again, as has adaptogen, in herbal medicine to characterize treatments that help patients feel better, but for which no scientific theory seems applicable.)

Our point here is that, while scientific medicine strives to establish clear-cut criteria for efficacy, it is important to find out how a patient defines it. A distinction increasingly made in scientific discussions between "efficacy" and "effectiveness" is useful. Efficacy describes treatment under ideal conditions (e.g., the controlled conditions of clinical trials), and effectiveness the everyday usage "in the field" where many more factors are at play. The latter range from relationships between practitioner and patient that can promote placebo responses (see below) to differences in bioavailability due to different diets. Ensuring effective concentrations of a product in the body is an issue generally considered in relationship to prescription drugs, but is being extended to dictary supplements.[59] It is important to appreciate that, although efficacy and effectiveness are commonly defined in different ways, the meaning we have given to the latter permeates complementary/alternative care. As one advocate of complementary/alternative medicine said, albeit discussing "efficacy": "one size doesn't fit all. You can take just about any natural health product of any variety, whether it's homeopathic, herbal, or in a vitamin form, and find that the amount that is appropriate for one group of individuals or one population is completely inappropriate for another."[60]

An appreciation of differences between efficacy and effectiveness can be helpful in evaluating clinical experience when it differs from research data. Unfortunately, we cannot explore this here beyond noting, as an example, that such an episode happened within therapeutic touch.[61] It can also help us in analyzing why research data often fails to be incorporated into practice.[62]

Placebo and Nocebo Effects

A complex issue facing complementary/alternative medicine is the charge that its effectiveness is "merely" a placebo effect. Although this often reflects ill-informed information or prejudices against complementary/alternative medicine, the widespread nature of the placebo response must be recognized.[63] The response (sometimes described as nonspecific effects) has been defined in countless ways, but most recognize a benefit from a treatment that, unknown to the patient, has no known physiological or pharmacological basis.

Placebos have a long history—by the nineteenth century they may well have been fairly widely administered to patients, at least to the worried well—but they only became a particularly prominent issue in the last fifty years or so because of their use as controls in randomized clinical trials. As these became the gold standard for testing drugs, it became increasingly apparent that placebo responses are commonplace in all manner of treatments.[64] To dismiss complementary/alternative care as "merely placebo" is to downplay a powerful force in therapy that can change the course of a patient's response to a disease quite dramatically.

Various ethical issues arise such as whether one should use placebos as controls in phase III trials (i.e., human trials) when existing, effective drugs could be used as controls.[65] Other concerns exist over the place of placebo in regular treatment; some practitioners argue that to use them consciously is unethical because this undermines the autonomy of the patient by deception, and reinforces the authority and power of the practitioner. Others, however, feel that many of the factors known to encourage the placebo response (e.g., empathy, trust) are hardly deception; indeed, some would say practitioners need to understand the virtues of the placebo effects and promote them.[66]

In this context, there is a professional responsibility to learn as much as possible about the placebo effect, which, in many ways, remains enigmatic. Presently, no clear answers have emerged from studies on why, for instance, some people are placebo responders and others are not. And why certain treatments (some technically sophisticated) prompt stronger placebo responses than others. Not surprisingly, no one theory has been generally accepted, and it may well be that there is not a single unitary explanation. However, it is generally appreciated that psychological influences are at play—e.g., belief in a treatment, and trust and hope considered under communication (see the section As a Communicator in Chapter 7).[67]

Complementary/alternative medicine is almost certainly no different from conventional medicine with regard to placebo responses; however, efforts to identify the placebo element in its treatments are of special importance because critics dismiss entire treatments as "merely placebo." Unfortunately there are few significant studies along the line of "Is evidence for homeopathy reproducible?" by D. Reilly and colleagues. They concluded that "homeopathy does more than placebo" in the treatment of hayfever and asthma.[68] A professional responsibility in considering such matters is to recognize patients' beliefs and the respect they demand. This is especially significant when one considers that inert or active treatments can not only produce placebo effects, but also negative outcomes (nocebo actions). The latter is a possibility whenever a patient *expects* a treatment to fail, has knowledge of side effects of a medication for which a placebo is substituted, or generally anticipates a negative outcome (possibly fostered by a practitioner's attitudes). Hopelessness, for example, has been associated with increasing the incidence and mortality in ischemic heart disease. This overall negative response (of which voodoo death is often given as an example) is sometimes contrasted with negative "side effects" (e.g., a new problem such as a skin rash) following the administration of a placebo.[69] Some observers suggest that nocebo responses are less likely in complementary/alternative than conventional care, but vigilance is always needed, especially when a patient arrives as a "last resort" with high hopes because everything else has failed.

NOTES

1. See D. M. Studdert, D. M. Eisenberg, F. H. Miller, D. A. Kurto, T. J. Kaptchuck, and T. A. Brennan, "Medical Malpractice Implications of Alternative Medicine," *JAMA*, 1998; 280, 1610-1618; I. Kennedy and A. Grubb, *Medical Law*, London: Butterworths, 1994, pp. 452-462; J. Stone and J. Matthews, *Complementary Medicine and the Law*, Oxford: Oxford University Press, 1996, p. 166.

2. C. Feasby, "Determining Standard of Care in Alternative Contexts," *Health Law Journal*, 1997; 5, 45-65.

3. For discussion of the United States: M. H. Cohen, *Complementary and Alternative Medicine: Legal Boundaries and Regulatory Perspectives*, Baltimore: Johns Hopkins Press, 1998, pp. 64-66.

4. For general discussion on practice guidelines for complementary/alternative medicine, Practice and Policy Guidelines Panel, National Institutes of Health Office of Alternative Medicine, "Clinical Practice Guidelines in Complementary and Alternative Medicine, An Analysis of Opportunities and Obstacles," *Archives of Family Medicine*, 1997; 6, 149-154. The situation described has changed relatively little in the early 2000s.

5. The national chiropractic guidelines in the United States are available from the American Chiropractic Association.

6. See book review by J. Goodman on "The Therapeutic Relationship in Complementary Health Care," *Complementary Therapies in Medicine*, 1998; 6, 224-225.

7. A. Avis, "When Is an Aromatherapist Not an Aromatherapist?" *Complementary Therapies in Medicine*, 1997; 7, 116-118.

8. Studdert et al., "Medical Malpractice."

9. Ibid.

10. G. Dukes, M. Mildred, B. Swartz, *Responsibility for Drug-Induced Injury: A Reference Book for Lawyers, the Health Professions and Manufacturers*, Amsterdam: IOS Press, 1998, p. 447.

11. Studdert et al., "Medical Malpractice."

12. J. Downie and T. Caulfield, eds., *Canadian Health Law and Policy*, Markham: Butterworths, 1999, p. 80.

13. For example, House of Commons Standing Committee on Health Minutes, March 25, 1998, p. 35.

14. Adapted from W. B. Jonas, "Safety in Complementary Medicine," in E. Ernst, ed., *Complementary Medicine: An Objective Appraisal,* Oxford: Butterworth-Heineman, 1996, pp. 126-149.

15. See H. A. Baer, "The Holistic Health Movement in the San Francisco Area: Some Preliminary Observations," *Social Science and Medicine,* 1998; 47, 1495-1501.

16. Comments in lecture by A. J. Romm, August 5, 1999, American Herb Guild Annual Meeting. Such an argument sidesteps the difficult issue of quality of the recording devices and the ideal circumstances under which blood pressure should be measured. Advice is sometimes given on how to avoid the language of diagnosis. Compare "The right to practise herbology, legal history and basis," from the Rocky Mountain Herbal Institute, <http://www.rmhiherbal.org/a/f.ahr3.rights.html> (accessed September 2001).

17. "A Comparative Evaluation of Diagnostic Systems Used in Herbal Medicine," <http://www.acupuncture.com/Diagnosis/CompDiag.htm> (accessed September 2001).

18. This list was appended to a 1998 Canadian definition of natural health products as substances or combinations for the purpose of maintaining or improving health and treating or preventing diseases/conditions. (Advisory Panel on Natural Health Products). The United States definition covers plant extracts, enzymes, vitamins, minerals and hormonal products available to the consumer without prescription; also included in a definition are such considerations as not being a conventional food.

19. One of the most recent warnings: F. M. Keane, S. E. Munn, A. W. P. du Vivier, N. F. Taylor, and E. M. Higgins, "Analysis of Chinese Herbal Creams Prescribed for Dermatological Conditions," *BMJ,* 1999; 318, 563-564. The article closed with a note on trends toward new controls in Britain.

20. Editorial: M. Angell and J. P. Kassirer: "Alternative Medicine—The Risks of Untested and Unregulated Remedies," *New England Journal of Medicine,* 1998, 339, 839-841.

21. See J. Barnes, S. Y. Mills, N. C. Abbott, M. Willoughby, and E. Ernst, "Different Standards for Reporting ADRs for Herbal Remedies and Conventional OTC Medicines: Face-to-Face Interviews with 515 Users of Herbal Medicines," *Pharmaceutical Journal,* 1998; 261, R21. Also J. Barnes, S.Y. Mills, M. Willoughby, and E. Ernst, "Different Standards for Reporting ADRs for Herbal Remedies and Conventional OTC Medicines: Face to Face Interviews with 515 Users of Herbal Remedies," *British Journal Clinical Pharmacy,* 1998; 45, 496-500.

22. Compare E. Ernst, "Second Thoughts About Safety of St. John's Wort," *Lancet,* 1999; 354, 2014-2016; also subsequent correspondence on this article, *Lancet* 2000; 355, 576-577. There is an increasing literature on herb-prescription drug incompatibilities. For example, from naturopathic physician F. Brinker, *Herb Contradictions and Drug Interactions*: *With Appendices Addressing Specific Conditions and Medicines,* Sandy, OR: Eclectic Medical Publishers, 1998. Various efforts continue to be made to develop national reporting systems. For a recent failure in the United Kingdom, "Healing Online Pioneers Online 'YellowCard' System," <http://www.healingonline.co.uk/tour/tour8.htm> (accessed January 2000, no longer available).

23. A. J. Vickers, R. W. Rees, and A. Robin, "Advice Given by Health Food Shops: Is It Clinically Safe? *Journal of the Royal College of Physicians of London,* 1998; 32, 426-428; also, editorial, E. Ernst, "Health Food Shops, Risks of Complementary Medicine, and Ethical Standards of Research, *Journal of the Royal College of Physicians of London,* 1998; 32, p. 399. The same concerns exist in North America.

24. *Maclean's,* 1998; September 21, 70-71; The case took on a life of its own. In 1999, the Canoe Health News continued the attack on chiropractic fueled by relatives of two women who died following chiropractic treatment: <http://www.canoe.ca/ chiro/york> (accessed December 1999, no longer available). See, too, M. M. De Roberts, "Chiropractic Goes to University," *The Scientific Review of Alternative Medicine,* 1998; 2, 49-54.

25. See review, T. J. Kaptchuk and D. M. Eisenberg, "Chiropractic Origins, Controversies, and Contributions," *Archives of Internal Medicine,* 1998; 158, 2215-2224.

26. For a still useful review of concerns over acupuncture: E. Ernst, "Acupuncture: Safety First," *BMJ,* 1997; 314, 1362; for aromatherapy, see J. Barnes, "Complementary Medicine Aromatherapy," *Pharmaceutical Journal,* 1998; 260, 862-867; for a sense of mounting concerns, W. C. Abbott, M. Hill, J. Barnes, P. G. Hourigan, and E. Ernst, "Uncovering Suspected Adverse Effects of Complementary and Alternative Medicine," *International Journal of Risk and Safety in Medicine,* 1998; 11, 99-106.

27. The issue of prayer has many ramifications for interesting discussion, G. S. Neeley, "Legal and Ethical Dilemmas Surrounding Prayer As a Method of Alternative Healing for Children," in J. M. Humber and R. F. Almeder, eds., *Alternative Medicine and Ethics,* Totowa, NJ: Humana Press, 1998, pp. 165-194.

28. K. D. Phillips, "Statutory Regulation Is Essential," *BMJ,* 1996; 313, 882; another report, "Acupuncture Patients Stripped and Blindfolded," *The Medical Post,* 1997; 33, 43.

29. Stone and Matthews, *Complementary Medicine and the Law,* Oxford: Oxford University Press, 1996, p. 201.

30. Ibid., p. 173.

31. E. Ernst, "Over-the-Counter Complementary Remedies for Arthritis," *Pharmaceutical Journal,* 1998; 260, 830-831.

32. See W. B. Jonas, "Safety in Homeopathy," in E. Ernst and E. G. Hahn, eds., *Homeopathy: A Critical Appraisal,* Oxford: Butterworth-Heinemann, 1998, pp. 130-135.

33. Compare E. Ernst, "Direct Risks Associated with Complementary Therapies," in E. Ernst, ed., *Complementary Medicine: An Objective Appraisal,* Oxford: Butterworth-Heinemann, 1996, pp. 112-125.

34. W. B. Jonas, "Safety in Complementary Medicine," in E. Ernst, ed., *Complementary Medicine: An Objective Appraisal,* Oxford: Butterworth-Heinemann, 1996, p. 126-149. See also W. B. Jonas and E. Ernst, "The Safety of Homeopathy," in W. B. Jonas and J. S. Levin, eds., *Essentials of Complementary Medicine,* Philadelphia: Lippincott, Williams and Wilkins, 1999, pp. 167-171.

35. House of Commons Standing Committee on Health Minutes, May 14, 1998, p. 9.

36. Over-the-counter strengths can be to 12C, 30C, an exception might be 200C arnica.

37. House of Commons Standing Committee on Health Minutes, May 13, 1998, p. 11. The statement was, in fact, made as Chair of the Advisory Panel on Natural Health Products, when defining "reasonable evidence" that could be used in support of the safety of a natural health product.

38. Ibid., February 3, 1998, p. 14, testimony of W. LeValley.

39. Quoted in M. McGuffin, C. Hobbs, R. Upton, and A. Goldberg, eds, *American Herbal Products Association Botanical Safety Handbook,* Boca Raton, FL: CRC Press, 1997, introduction.

40. C, Vincent and A. Furnham, *Complementary Medicine: A Research Perspective,* New York: Wiley, 1997, p. 135.

41. Much controversy surrounds the scholarship of historian J. M. Riddle who argues that ancient uses of many plant medicines, once forgotten, have been rediscovered in modern times. However, questions arise about the relevance of changing terminology of symptoms, misinterpretations of past terminology, modes of administration of products, size of doses, and much more. For an example of Riddle's work: "Historical Data As an Aid in Pharmaceutical Prospecting and Drug Safety Determination," *Journal of Alternative and Complementary Medicine,* 1999; 5(2), 195-201. Riddle notes that several products presently sold in health stores were historically used as abortifacients. "Use of these products should be interdicted for pregnant women, even if other laboratory data is unavailable" (p. 200).

42. Quoted by R. Porter in S. Lock, L. A. Reynolds, and E. M. Tansey, eds., *Ashes to Ashes: The History of Smoking and Health,* Amsterdam: Rodopi, 1998, p. 222.

43. For use of phrase "test of time" with comments: E. Ernst and J. Barnes, "Methodological Approaches to Investigating the Safety of Complementary Medicine," *Complementary Therapies in Medicine,* 1998; 6, 115-121. Their emphasis is that conditions of usage are commonly much different nowadays than in the past.

44. Compare J. M. Riddle, *Eve's Herbs: A History of Contraception and Abortion in the West,* Cambridge: Harvard University Press, 1997, who emphasizes loss of information on abortion and birth control. As he says, there was a "divorce of information about birth control and modern 'professional' medicine" (p. 203). Riddle's views, however, do not go unchallenged.

45. The Digitalis Investigation Group, "The Effect of Digoxin on Mortality and Morbidity in Patients with Heart Failure," *New England Journal of Medicine,* 1997; 336(8), 525-533.

46. House of Commons Standing Committee on Health Minutes, March 17, 1998, pp. 40-41. In the same vein the long history of blood-letting to treat countless conditions—now widely considered as valueless (except for at least one condition)—is more commonly cited.

47. M. Packer, "End of the Oldest Controversy in Medicine: Are We Ready to Conclude the Debate on Digitalis?" *New England Journal of Medicine* 1997; 336(8), 575-576.

48. For an example of negative media publicity, digitalis and plantain, see U.S. Food and Drug Administration warning June 12, 1997. Compare "Herbal remedy

rifts unsettling to industry. Drug manufacturers trade allegations in competitive market short on regulations," *The Globe and Mail*, March 12, 1999, p. A3.

49. Quote from M. Blumenthal, meeting report, *Environmental Health Perspectives*, 1998; 106, A590-A592.

50. For examples of self-regulation: M. McGuffin, "Self-Regulatory Initiatives by the Herbal Industry," *HerbalGram*, 2000, No. 48, 42-43.

51. The survey was of preparations available in Canada, but analogous situations occur in the United States and elsewhere. See also, D. V. C. Awang, "Feverfew Effective in Migraine Prevention," *HerbalGram*, 1998, No. 42, 18.

52. Compare D. V. C. Awang, "Prescribing Therapeutic Feverfew (*Tanacetum parthenium* (L.) Schultz Bip., syn *Chrysanthemum parthenium* (L.) Bernh.)," *Integrative Medicine*, 1998; 1, 11-13.

53. For example, F. Brinker, "Variations in Effective Botanical Products," *HerbalGram*, 1999; No. 46(Spring), 35-50.

54. C. Minter, "Standardising Herbal Medicine," *Journal of the Australian Traditional-Medicine Society*, 1997; 3(2), 71.

55. House of Commons Standing Committe on Health Minutes, February 19, 1998, p. 30.

56. Ibid., March 10, 1998, p. 28.

57. For example, M. Pedersen, *Nutritional Herbology*, Bountiful: Pedersen Publishing, 1989.

58. Making patients feel better has become part of the language of alternative medicine; as an example House of Commons Standing Committee on Health (Canada), *Natural Health Products: A New Vision*, 1998, section 4D.

59. "Bioavailability of Dietary Supplements," *Pharmaceutical Journal*, 2000; 264, 304-305.

60. House of Commons Standing Committee on Health Minutes, February 5, 1998.

61. An interesting 1998 study found that practitioners could not accurately discern the presence or absence of a "human energy field." L. Rosa, E. Rosa, L. Sarner, and S. Barrett, "A Close Look at Therapeutic Touch," *JAMA*, 1998; 279, 1005-1010. This brought much criticism of the methodology, see *JAMA*, 1998; 280, 1905-1908. More recent reviews of research call for further research to clarify discordant results, e.g., P. Winstead-Fry and J. Kijek, "An Integrative Review and Meta-Analysis of Therapeutic Touch Research," *Alternative Therapies in Health and Medicine*, 1999; 5(6), 58-67.

62. For some discussion of issues: G. T. Lewith, "The Use and Abuse of Evidence-Based Medicine: an Example from General Practice," in E. Ernst, ed., *Complementary Medicine: An Objective Appraisal*, Oxford: Butterworth-Heinemann, 1996, pp. 106-111.

63. Compare A. K. Shapiro and E. Shapiro, *The Powerful Placebo: From Ancient Priest to Modern Physician*, Baltimore: Johns Hopkins University Press, 1997.

64. For background, A. J. M. de Craen, T. J. Kaptchuk, J. G. Tijssen, and J. Kleijnen, "Placebos and Placebo Effects in Medicine: Historical Overview," *Journal of the Royal Society of Medicine*, 1999; 92, 511-515. T. J. Kaptchuk, "In-

tentional Ignorance: A History of Blind Assessment and Placebo Controls in Medicine," *Bulletin of the History of Medicine,* 1998; 72, 389-433.

65. For example, F. Garcia-Alonso, E. Guallar, O. M. Bakke, and X. Carné, "Use and Abuse of Placebo in Phase III Trials," *European Journal of Clinical Pharmacology,* 1998; 54, 101-105.

66. For example, N. Biller, "The Placebo Effect: Mocking or Mirroring Medicine," *Perspectives in Biology and Medicine,* 1999; 42, 398-401.

67. de Craen et al., "Placebos and Placebo Effects in Medicine." Kaptchuk, "Intentional Ignorance."

68. *Lancet,* 1994; 344, 1601-1606. Also D. Reilly, "Is Homeopathy a Placebo Response? What If It Is? What If It Is Not?" in E. Ernst and E. G. Hahn, eds., *Homeopathy: A Critical Appraisal,* Oxford: Butterworth-Heinemann, 1998, pp. 118-129. This adds interest to the fact that nineteenth-century homeopathy contributed to the use of the placebo as a control in clinical trials, M. E. Dean, "A Homeopathic Origin for Placebo Controls: 'An Invaluable Gift of God,'" *Alternative Therapies in Health and Medicine,* 2000; 6, 58-66.

69. See R. A. Hahn, "The Nocebo Phenomenon: Concept, Evidence, and Implications for Public Health," *Preventive Medicine,* 1997; 26, 607-611.

Chapter 5

Regulation by Legislation or Self-Regulation?

Given the issues raised so far (for instance, appropriate standards of care, who should make diagnoses, and disagreements over potential toxicity of many dietary supplements), it is not surprising that countless, contentious debates have arisen over what should or should not be legislated, what should be self-regulated, and the possible balance between the two. The debates—many stirred by government scrutiny, already mentioned—mostly focus on appropriate controls over, for example, on herbal remedies and on the licensing of practitioners by statutory legislation rather than "certification" through an organization of practitioners. The credibility of such certification depends, of course, on the credibility of the organization, how representative it is, and the standards employed. In fact, most of the 1990s debate was on the safety of herbs when sold as dietary supplements. This is discussed first in this section that briefly examines various substantial issues, especially for complementary/alternative medicine.

DIETARY SUPPLEMENTS AND REGULATIONS: DIVERSE ATTITUDES

The two health care cultures we have discussed are particularly conspicuous in debates on dietary supplements. On the one side, medical organizations, public health experts, and regulators believe that supplements should be treated as medicines, not foods, and that the three pillars of safety, quality, and efficacy are needed to protect the public. On the other side, there is vigorous opposition to controls from those who demand freedom of choice in health care. At the heart of the dichotomy is the matter of public interest versus patient autonomy, coupled with charges of self-serving interests. Should regulation policies be as minimal as possible—implemented only when they are shown to be necessary to protect public health—or should they protect the public from *possible* dangers and abuse by patients? The latter can mean, for example, accepting that dosages of vitamins and minerals—e.g., above the Recommended Daily Allowance—be classified as medicines as is done in France and Spain.[1]

Public policy decisions are commonly compromises, which have the potential to satisfy no one. Recent legislation offers much to consider. Striking is the Dietary Supplement Health and Education Act (DSHEA) of the United States enacted in 1994, which arose out of strong grassroots support for changing the legislation and allowing more consumer choice. In a dramatic departure from previous regulations, the new Act established that dietary supplements can be marketed without prior approval of the U.S. Food and Drug Administration (FDA). The latter can only withdraw unsafe products after they have been marketed, the initial determination of safety resting with the manufacturer. When the full story of the Act and its impact is written, much will be said about the subsequent public confusion and continuing tussles with the FDA, especially over health (structure/ function) claims allowed by the Act, and the confusion between dietary supplements and medicinal herbs. As one health information network has said (1998), "the distinction between drugs and dietary supplements recently has become more and more confusing for consumers."[2] Clearly all practitioners have a responsibility to help in this area, to evaluate the rampant commercialism, clinical, and other data. Such guidance will be needed all the more if the late 1990s trend to market dietary supplements as beverages, spreads, and other "non-pill" dosage forms becomes more widespread.[3]

A Canadian example of compromise legislation, in the form of a third *regulatory* category for Natural Health Products distinct from "foods" or "drugs," allows greater government control of dietary supplements than in the United States.[4] Only time will tell whether many concerns associated with the compromise will be resolved.[5] It is of particular interest that another regulatory model, namely a category of "Traditional Medicines," established in Canada in the mid-1990s, may or may not be continued. Indeed this model utilized in many countries (e.g., France, Belgium, and Switzerland)—which recognizes both safety considerations and traditional uses on labels—appears to be an "honest" way of proceeding so long as the historical record is assessed critically (see previous chapter). It was being discussed during the time of the establishment of DSHEA in the United States, but was pushed to one side.[6] Even if the category disappears, the approach deserves professional consideration in any discussion on public safety.

We do not have space to discuss the trends toward greater regulation and standardization of herbal products that are emerging from the European Union where, in the early 2000s, getting agreement from country to country continued to be difficult. However, the trend is important. Many feel fairly certain that there will be general acceptance that only products meeting "requirements on safety and *efficacy* by either specific bibliographic reference and/or coverage through monographs or core SPCs [summaries of product characteristics] and/or clinical trials according to an appropriate model will be able to gain European-wide access."[7] This may include traditional uses for some herbs.

The tensions over dietary supplement regulation prompt considerations about professional regulation in general. Should the goal of complementary/alternative medicine be self-regulation or some balance between statutory and self-regulation? Should statutory regulation, such as suggested in a proposed Acupuncture Act, extend to telling practitioners that they should not inform patients that acupuncture cures disease.[8]

STATUTORY REGULATION OR SELF-REGULATION?

Although self-regulation—considered a key characteristic of any profession—is the policy of complementary/alternative medical organizations on both sides of the Atlantic, it must be seen in the context that society has introduced so many controls that, today, mainstream health professions are often viewed as only quasi-self-regulating. Legislation, for instance, limits many physician roles and sets regulatory frameworks for licensing and for disciplinary measures. We are being reminded constantly that what is left of self-regulation in the health professions needs continuous attention.[9] As the British medical profession was reminded in 1997 by the President of the General Medical Council, it is "failing to make self-regulation demonstrably effective and responsive" amid "criticisms that we are not addressing the widespread [public] dissatisfaction with the attitude of some doctors, including their paternalism and poor communication with both patients and colleagues."[10]

Given the history of the conventional medical profession, many ask how can one expect complementary/alternative practitioners—who frequently do not belong to well-established and stable organizations—to maintain, without legislative boundaries, uniform educational and disciplinary standards.[11] Can professional ethics alone ensure appropriate self-regulated standards of education, safety, quality, and efficacy? Or is statutory licensure (see Licensing, later in this chapter) an essential framework for professional standards? The answers to such questions, to which polarized responses can be found within complementary/alternative medicine, may well be at the heart of its long-term future as a professional force in health care.

Those who believe that current goals of unregulated complementary/alternative practitioners should be to pursue self-regulation offer different strategies in bringing this about. Up front, however, is adherence to appropriate codes of ethics and standards of education that can withstand public scrutiny. For instance, Stone and Matthews, when discussing the British scene, argue that "substantive ethical teaching must be a part of all practitioners' training." Stone adds that any "rush toward statutory regulation as opposed to professionalisation is misguided," that legislation is a straitjacket, and that "most therapies should continue working toward accreditation and the development of national standards of training and competence."[12] The best safeguards for the public are high levels of competence, ensured through high standards of training and supervision.

The only useful function that statutory regulation, according to Stone and Mathews, provides over voluntary regulation is the ability to protect a professional title by making it illegal for nonregistered practitioners to use that title. On the other hand, the authors acknowledge difficulties in that "none of the existing complementary codes of ethics in Britain [and by implication elsewhere] truly identify what is required of practitioners in order to act ethically."[13] Furthermore, although the suggestion that the onus should be on patients to verify a practitioner's credentials before entering a therapeutic relationship is sound advice, this is onerous for patients in the absence of national standards, even when registers of practitioners are maintained by organizations.

It is beyond the scope of this volume to consider specific self-regulatory models, except for a couple of points. While significant progress has occurred in Britain in improving standards through self-regulation by national bodies, developing national, as opposed to state or provincial, standards is difficult to attain in North America.[14] Suggestions are made that unionization—generally an anathema to professionalism—may be one consideration. Indeed, for other reasons, it is now being considered by many physicians in the United States who are concerned with the ever-growing bureaucracy in health care. In Quebec, a noteworthy example of self-regulation has occurred through unionization of complementary/alternative care. For instance, many alternative practitioners belong to the Fédération des Professionels. Acupuncturists joined the federation in 1988, followed by homeopaths (1989), naturopaths (1995), and osteopaths (1996). However, questions must be raised about the standards for registration, if only because a conflict of interest exists between the needs of unions to attract as large a membership as possible and the need to maintain high standards.

EDUCATION

Complementary/Alternative Medicine: The General Scene

Quality educational institutions must have a key role in any development of professional standards in complementary/alternative medicine. Unfortunately, their current diversity, with different standards and accreditation bodies in virtually all areas of complementary/alternative care, is problematic. In many ways, the current scene parallels private nineteenth-century conventional medical schools that faced the same dilemmas of trying to find agreement on the appropriate balance between scientific (or theoretical) and clinical training, and on how to improve standards amid disagreements and infighting among interested parties.[15] This, was, in fact, a stage in professionalization that took what might be called diploma level standards in some schools to university and postgraduate qualifications. Whether the same will happen to complementary/alternative medicine remains debatable.

Generally speaking, despite the disparate scene (with at least some premier schools in such key modalities as acupuncture, chiropractic, homeopathy, and naturopathy), complementary/alternative medical education received relatively little scrutiny from the general public during the 1980s to 1990s. Indeed, in North America more interest existed in how many medical schools were teaching alternative medicine.[16] However, with growing numbers of nonmedically licensed practitioners, public concerns over competency and the attendant difficulty of assessing qualifications were becoming increasingly evident by 2000.

One consequence of public concerns is for colleges and universities (always looking for new sources of revenue) to offer new courses. Britain is a noteworthy example; already by 1998, a trend was emerging for complementary/alternative medicine education to be incorporated into the British university system. "Degree, diploma and certificate courses in acupuncture, homeopathy, therapeutic massage, herbal medicine and 'complementary therapies' etc., are now available, in addition to the more established courses of chiropractic and osteopathy."[17] One particularly significant consequence is that universities will produce practitioners who will "acquire academic qualifications and an understanding of research methodology."

Analogous trends were emerging in North America by 2000, although more to sensitize students in general to complementary/alternative care rather than to train and educate practitioners. This may change if vigorous opposition from university faculty—e.g., chiropractic in places—to developing courses for practitioners is defeated.[18] Indeed, complementary/alternative medical organizations must consider whether existing public colleges and universities should replace private, for-profit schools if the latter fail to develop consistent standards. Nowhere is the issue of chaotic standards better illustrated than in Toronto, which entered the new millennium with intense competition and infighting between at least eight schools of homeopathy. Their lengths of education, and accreditation or support range widely. Total course hours vary from 728 to 3,045.[19] Thirteen accreditation bodies or institutions are listed by the schools, but no two have the same list, and some give none.[20] Unlike mainstream medicine, there are no universally accepted national accreditation organizations; moreover, the accreditation standards of the bodies that exist are virtually inaccessible to the general public or even to practitioners. Indeed, there are substantial professional disagreements over standards, even where they exist. A case in point is whether standards for acupuncture should cover both traditional and modern practices.

Curricula Content and Continuing Education

This is not the place to offer any detailed comment on course content. However, we notice three topics that tend to be contentious in order to prime discussion on standards. The first is how much basic science (e.g., anatomy, physiology, and biochemistry) should be known by complementary/alternative practitioners, even if much of it seems irrelevant to their everyday practice. We have already raised the issue in noting the growing recognition among complementary/alternative practitioners that the same evaluation standards are needed as in mainstream medicine (see related discussion in Chapter 2). There is, too, the matter of integration (see corresponding section in Chapter 3) and the need for mutual understandings between all practitioners, particularly about diagnosis.

Although certain modalities and schools offer substantial basic science education, it needs to be emphasized that solid basic science knowledge may, for example,

1. aid a complementary/alternative practitioner's ability to understand the conventional medical treatment a patient may be having;
2. increase an "index of suspicion" of multisystem disease and of cases that should be referred to others;
3. help to recognize possible incompatibilities between two treatments; and
4. ensure that practitioners constantly evaluate research and the changing relationships between complementary/alternative care and medical science.

We suggest that basic science teaching must also cover the philosophy and methodology of science. In order for effective communication amid the different perspectives on science and complementary/alternative medicine, there needs to be common understanding of the various meanings given to, for example, observation, hypothesis, theory, experiment, and verification of experiments. We have noted, too, issues over the term reductionism and the way ideologies can shape arguments.

The second curriculum topic we notice is the subject of this volume, professional and ethical issues. Unfortunately, compared with mainstream medical and nursing education, these have generally received little or no formal classroom activity, though some premier complementary/alternative institutions are responding to some extent. Although we hope this volume, standing alone, serves as a sound introduction to relevant issues, the importance of classroom debate and discussion can be significant in developing skills of critical appraisal of ethical situations, and to lay firm foundations for complementary/alternative medicine's secure future.

Our third point relates to the growing general attention to continuing education. Indeed, this is now mandatory for continued registration for various medical specialties in North America. Although many hurdles exist to establish this widely in complementary/alternative care, it has to be looked at in the context of professional responsibility and even in tegration.

COMPLEMENTARY/ALTERNATIVE EDUCATION FOR MAINSTREAM PRACTITIONERS

A concern of many observers is the inadequacy of training of regular physicians in complementary/alternative medicine. In fact, despite the deep frustrations over the regulations of the Alberta College of Physicians and Surgeons (see discussion in Chapter 2), that College's general concerns with educational standards are justified. Although, for example, "modern" or Westernized acupuncture (sometimes called anatomical acupuncture) is now well established, published statements such as the following from a British physician may seem cavalier and certainly need careful assessment:

> The kind of acupuncture I practise is modern or non-traditional, and I teach it to doctors and physiotherapists in 2-day courses. These are both somewhat contentious matters, for some people maintain that the only "real" acupuncture is the traditional version and that it is impossible to learn anything worthwhile about the subject in a short course. However, I am unrepentant.[21]

One of the issues raised by such comments is whether condensed courses for those trained in Western anatomy and physiology lead to quality care. For instance, does acupuncture depend solely on using acupoints that are associated with specific symptoms (empirical practice), or is theoretical knowledge required that suggests the use of additional points to improve the level of care? Such matters deserve scientific and public debate, especially if it brings acupuncture into the mind-set of the reductionism of conventional medicine.

We do not have space to examine complementary/alternative education for nurses, but their ethic of care may well help to ensure that holistic approaches are sustained.

RESEARCH

We have discussed the growing appreciation within complementary/alternative medicine that it should be subjected to the same scientific scrutiny as mainstream medicine. This may need new research methodologies, and a critical appraisal of the view that "trial participants are regarded as members of an equivalence class, defined by the diagnosis, who all will be given a standard prescribed treatment" rather than individualized treatment.[22] We argue that leadership in research, both basic and clinical, should come, at least in part, from many more educational institutions for complementary/alternative medicine (supported by industry and foundations) than at present. Aside from widespread agreement on the need for further research, this would contribute to fulfilling educational responsibilities to train students to evaluate research critically.

This is not the place to discuss the growing literature, considered by others, on research and research methodology to evaluate complementary/alternative medicine.[23] Nor can we review the innumerable instances of fraud and fudging in medical scientific research that have been uncovered in recent years. However, we must mention that, nowadays, high ethical standards are demanded for all human investigation research. Mainstream medical research must be approved by an independent ethics review board. Moreover, mainline medical journals will only publish studies where such approval is documented. Presently, complementary/alternative clinical studies, especially when done in office settings, do not generally meet this requirement. Although participants may have given informed consent, an independent ethical review provides not only a check on safety, but also on the appropriateness of a study design. One difficulty for complementary/alternative practitioners is that they may not have ready access to such a review board, or, if they do, the board may be unfamiliar with the methodology to evaluate, say, homeopathy. A responsibility exists for complementary/alternative organizations to review closely such issues, all the more because of many concerns over the quality of research in their field.

LICENSING

The twenty-first century opened with considerable variation in statutory licensing between countries, and between the states and provinces across the United States and Canada, where some license a few modalities (e.g., acupuncture, massage) and others none. Partly because of such variation, some form of self-regulation (discussed earlier in this chapter) or statutory licensing had become a central issue in government and public scrutiny. Even in England and Scotland where, under common law, anyone has a right to practice medicine (so long as they do not use a title that implies they are licensed), there are calls for licensing to be introduced, as happened to chiropractic and osteopathy in the 1990s. Amid growing public demand for licensing lies particular interest in two "models," one Canadian and one U.S., on which we comment.

British Columbia and Ontario both have relatively new Health Professions Acts (called Regulated Health Professions Act [RHPA] in Ontario). These can be seen as having the potential to break down traditional hierarchies, at least that is part of the philosophy behind them as expressed by one authority on the Ontario Act who indicated that the "policy thrust underlying the Act—making more efficient use of all health professions without compromising public protection—is very different from the policy agenda underlying the statutes it has replaced."[24] Unlike the previous statutes, the Act would not necessarily limit consumer freedom of choice and would not stand in the way of creative utilization of individual health professionals. A further telling comment is that the new RHPA "would regulate every profession according to the same rules and thus exert a leveling influence across the elite, predominately male health professions and the lower rung, predominately female professions." In consequence, the regulation of acupuncture would, for instance, be no different from conventional medicine. As an example, British Columbia recently evaluated applications for Traditional Chinese Medicine to be designated a health profession, and accepted that licensing would be in the public interest and safety.

Central to the Canadian trends is maintaining the separateness, the integrity, of each modality. This contrasts with the potentially far-reaching Complementary and Alternative Health Freedom of Access Act of Minnesota, signed into law May 2000. This sets up a single new office to provide government oversight of a broad spectrum of unlicensed complementary/alternative practitioners. The office will receive consumer complaints, investigate them, and enforce a lengthy list of prohibitions to practice (e.g., conviction of fraud, false or misleading advertising, sexual contact with patients, and inability to practice "with reasonable safety. . . to clients"). The lengthy history of the passage of the Act is a classic instance of grassroots demands for choice challenging the status quo and establishment conservatism.[25]

Even from these brief notes on developments, it should be clear that significant issues are at stake. Although, as indicated already, there are good arguments for professional bodies regulating their own licensing, the trend is to have some form of statutory control, or a mix of the two. Although the particular form will rest with each jurisdiction, professional input is always needed in discussions on how best to balance public protection and patient choice.

DISCIPLINARY MEASURES

One further issue needs specific mention, namely, How do health professions discipline their members? After all, codes of ethics (see Part II) are much less useful if there are no mechanisms to enforce them. Indeed, disciplining is viewed as an important hallmark of self-regulation, especially as it can deprive a person of his or her livelihood for contravening standards established by the profession. Responsibilities exist with respect to justice, since the standards of evidence required for disciplining may not meet those required by a court of law.

Questions constantly arise whether physicians and the public are satisfied with the work of medical disciplinary boards? This is often tied to different views on the roles of boards. For instance, do they (or should they) represent the profession alone? How many lay members should be on a disciplinary board? In other words, to what extent do boards represent the public or more broadly the state? What should practitioners be disciplined for? Also, in North America, where licensing is a state and provincial matter, how can standards be made more and more equable from jurisdiction to jurisdiction so as to respond to public concerns about variations in standards?[26] Given all such questions, one can ask: Are current medical boards suitable models for complementary/alternative medicine? In fact, should disciplining be done by an independent board?[27] Professionalism demands careful consideration of such matters.

NOTES

1. P. Mason, "Regulation of Dietary Supplements—Time for a Change," *Pharmaceutical Journal,* 1998; 260, 528-530.

2. <http://www.heartinfo.com/news98/fdalabels5898htm> (accessed May, 1998, no longer available).

3. See L. Israelson, "Five Major Issues to Dominate Supplements Industry in 1999," *Natural Business,* 1999; January 13, no pagination.

4. The sense of compromise between those "who see protection of consumers as a paramount responsibility" and "members of the public who are informed consumers practicing self-care" becomes clear from the results of the deliberations of the House of Commons Standing Committee on Health Minutes.

5. Issues cover antiscience and beliefs that homeopathic preparations, traditional Chinese remedies, and vitamins and minerals do not belong in the same regulatory category. For some aspects, J. Chang, "Scientific Evaluation of Traditional Chinese Medicine Under DSHEA: A Conundrum," *The Journal of Alternative and Complementary Medicine,* 1999; 5, 181-189. For a grassroots medical backlash, B. Sibbald, "New Group Sets Sights on Herbal Medicines," *Canadian Medical Association Journal,* 1999; 161, 583.

6. For some discussion on traditional medicine models at the time: M. Blumenthal, "Regulatory Models for Approval of Botanicals As Traditional Medicines," in D. Eskinazi, ed., *Botanical Medicine: Efficacy, Quality Assurance, and Regulation,* Larchmont, NY: Liebert, 1999, pp. 205-212.

7. For discussion and quote, H. Cranz, "Regulation of Traditional Medicines: European Experience," in *Responsible Self-Medication: Recognizing Its Role in Total Health Care. Proceedings of the World Self-Medication Industry (WSMI), 3rd Asia Pacific Regional Conference,* Kuala Lumpur, Malaysia, 1998, pp. 84-88. See also M. McIntyre, "Protecting the Availability of Herbal Medicines," *The Journal of Alternative and Complementary Medicine,* 1999; 5, 109-110, and "Alternative Licensing for Herbal Medicine-Like Products in the European Union," *The Journal of Alternative and Complementary Medicine,* 1999, 5, 110-113.

A specific issue of professional concern to complementary/alternative practitioners (as well as users) is the work of the Codex Alimentarius, the International Commission charged with bringing international food standards into being. Much opposition states that the Codex will lead to the banning of countless dietary supplements. For a sense of the extensive concerns with the Codex on the Internet see for example, <http://www.therapure.com/codex.htm> (accessed September 2001).

8. From the Ontario Associates of Acupuncture and Traditional Chinese Medicine, February 2000, p. 7. The proposed new Act talks of approval by a board, but standards of accreditation are not made clear. We add here that one form of regulation rarely discussed is city bylaws. It is noteworthy that a Toronto bylaw calls for an annual license fee and requires practitioners to submit evidence of education achievement, and sanitary conditions with the Toronto Licensing Commission, which also limits services.

9. For example, J. N. Johnson, "Making Self-Regulation Credible Through Bench-Marking, Peer Review, Appraisal, and Management," *BMJ,* 1998; 316, 1847-1848.

10. D. Irvine, "The Performance of Doctors. I: Professionalism and Self-Regulation in a Changing World," *BMJ,* 1997; 314, 1540-1542.

11. J. Stone and J. Matthews, *Complementary Medicine and the Law,* Oxford: Oxford University Press, 1996, p. 206.

12. Stone and Matthews, *Complementary Medicine and the Law,* p. 208; J. Stone, "Regulating Complementary Medicine: Should Aim for Standards Not Status," *BMJ,* 1996; 312, 1492-1493.

13. Stone and Matthews, *Complementary Medicine and the Law,* p. 208.

14. The issue is particularly evident in Canada where the administration of the Canada Health Act is considered a sovereign issue for the provinces.

15. For context, K. M. Ludmerer, *Learning to Heal: The Development of American Medical Education,* New York: Basic Books, 1985, e.g., p. 3.

16. See, for instance, M. S. Wetzel, D. M. Eisenberg, and T. D. Kaptchuk, "Courses Involving Complementary and Alternative Medicine at U.S. Medical Schools," *JAMA,* 1998; 280, 784-787. This was followed by interesting correspondence reflecting the diversity of attitudes (*JAMA,* 1999; 281, 609-611), but with support for the five guidelines for alternative medicine education in medical schools with emphasis on critical appraisal and communication with alternative health care clinicians and patients. On the other hand, the correspondence reveals outrage that schools are affected by "political correctness" of the times and that they should be resistant to "fads and fakirs." "We, as physicians, must be the last bastion of science in this sea of pseudoscience that is flooding the airwaves and cyberspace." See also, "Medical Schools Failing to Take 'Skeptical' View of Alt. Med," *The Medical Post,* 1999; 35 (March 23), 34. Also, for lay interest in medical schools, "The Changing Face of Canadian Medical Schools," *Health Naturally,* 1997, December/January, 24-25; for additional information, J. Ruedy, D. M. Kaufman, and H. MacLoed, "Alternative and Complementary Medicine in Canadian Medical Schools: A Survey," *Canadian Medical Association Journal,* 1999; 160, 816-817.

17. Compare D. Morgan, H. Glanville, S. Mars, and V. Nathanson, "Education and Training in Complementary and Alternative Medicine: Postal Survey of U.K. Universities, Medical Schools and Faculties of Nurse Education," *Complementary Therapies in Medicine,* 1998; 6, 64-70.

18. As one example, see T. Johnson, "Angry Scientists Fight University's Attempt to Affiliate with Chiropractic College," *Canadian Medical Association Journal,* 1999; 160, 99-100 [about York University in Toronto]. See also Y. Y. Yip, "New Age Medicine Meets Western Science," *University Affairs,* 1999 (October), 16-19.

19. Information from calendars of the following homeopathic schools in Toronto, though hours not given for many schools: British Institute of Homeopathy, Canada, Canadian Academy of Homeopathy, Canadian College of Classical Homeopathy, Canadian College of Homeopathy (now Canadian College of Natural Healing), Hahnemann College of Homeopathy Canadian Campus, Hahnemannian

College of Classical Homeopathy (Canadian College of Classical Homeopathy), Homeopathic College of Canada, Toronto School of Homeopathic Medicine Ltd.

20. The list includes: Association of General Practitioners of Natural Medicine, British Faculty of Osteopathy, British Naturopath and Osteopathy Association, Canadian Association of Homeopathic Physicians (B.C.), Council of Homeopathic Education (for post-graduate training), Hahnemann College of Homeopathy (U.K.), Hahnemann College of Homeopathy (Canada), Hahnemannia Association of Classical Homeopathy (Canada), Homeopathic Medical Council of Canada, Manitoba Homeopathic Association, Ontario Homeopathic Association, Society for Complementary Medicine, United Kingdom Homeopathic Medical Association.

21. A. Campbell, "A Doctor's View of Acupuncture: Traditional Chinese Theories Are Unnecessary," *Complementary Therapies in Medicine,* 1998; 6, 152-155.

22. A. Margolin, S. K. Avants, and D. Kleber, "Investigating Alternative Medicine Therapies in Randomized Controlled Trials," *JAMA,* 1998; 280, 1626-1628.

23. For example, K. Linde and W. B. Jonas, "Evaluating Complementary and Alternative Medicine: The Balance of Rigor and Relevance," in W. B. Jonas and J. S. Levin, eds., *Essentials of Complementary and Alternative Medicine,* Philadelphia: Lippincott Williams and Wilkins, 1999, pp. 57-87.

24. L. S. Bohnen, *Regulated Health Professions Act: A Practical Guide,* Aurora: Canada Law Book, 1994, pp. v, 2.

25. Statute 146A. For context compare literature from Minnesota Natural Health Legal Reform Project and <www.minnesotanaturalhealth.org> (accessed September 2000).

26. As an instance of the issues, in 1996 the U.S.-based Public Citizen's Health Research Group stated that statistics indicate that some state medical boards (U.S.) are far less aggressive in disciplining doctors than others. It was reported that some states are 10 times more likely to mete out punishments for offenses ranging from insurance fraud to sexual misconduct to incompetence. For continuing concern of the group about the disciplining of physicians, see <http://www.citizen.org/hrg> (accessed September 2001).

27. A publication available from the National Acupuncture Foundation, 1718 M. Street, Suite 195, Washington, DC, sets out a summary of the state laws pertaining to acupuncture. As an example of variations, acupuncture falls under the jurisdiction of Alberta Health and Wellness/Health Discipline's Board which is the Provincial Department of Health. The Health Discipline's Board establishes the educational requirements and approves programs of study in acupuncture. In Quebec, on the other hand, the regulating body for non-MD acupuncturists is the Order of Acupuncturists.

PART II: PROFESSIONALISM

Chapter 6

Professionalism: Many Faces

INTRODUCTION: DIVERSE VIEWS

What does it mean to be a professional? Part I has provided a sense of many issues to be considered. Here we explore more the professional/ethical framework. Accordingly we focus on topics relevant to the steps for consideration in evaluating any ethical dilemma. For convenience we repeat the steps here:

1. The data or "facts" (scientific, clinical, legal, and sociocultural
2. A patient's beliefs, concepts, and ideologies about health and disease and how these may differ from mainstream views
3. A practitioner's personal values, attitudes (including to ethics), and biases that may affect decision making
4. Ethical theories and codes of ethics that guide one's thinking
5. How best to negotiate, with sensitivity, ethical decisions with a patient and his or her family, as well as with colleagues.

We also consider how professionalism is defined or identified by the profession itself and by outsiders, specifically sociologists and the general public. In doing so, we must remember that change is always happening. Many observers of health care argue that the nature of professionalism changed in the late twentieth century. Students, in particular, should wonder about this continuing during their professional lives, and what contribution they might make.

Much of our discussion of professionalism emerges from a consideration of mainstream medicine, which is often viewed as a "model" for the study of professionalism.[1] However, the issues we raise need to be evaluated by complementary/alternative practitioners, indeed by everyone offering health care. First, we should notice that, increasingly during the 1990s physicians saw "genuine medical professionalism in peril"; American Bernard Lown comments (1996) on an apparent erosion of professional values in medicine:

> Medicine's profound crisis, I believe, is only partially related to ballooning costs, for the problem is far deeper than economics. In my view, the basic reason is that medicine has lost its way, if not its soul. An unwritten covenant between doctor and patient, hallowed over several millennia, is being broken.[2]

In the United Kingdom, calls exist for a new professionalism.[3] As part of this and amid public concerns about medical standards, the General Medical Council has made clear (1998) that physicians' "standards" are a public issue. Medicine needs to be "open" to scrutiny. British physicians are warned: "If serious problems arise which call your registration [medical license] into question, these are the standards [made public] against which you will be judged."[4] Clearly, a more rigorous approach to enforcing ethical standards than hitherto emerged in the 1990s.

Calls also exist in mainstream medicine for formal training in professionalism.[5] Many doubt that "inheriting" professionalism from parents who were physicians, or through the influence of other role models is any longer sufficient. In fact, various reasons have been put forth to account for the erosion of such traditional professional values as compassion, service, and integrity. Particular worries exist, especially in the United States, over the impact of commercialism, the ideology of free markets, corporate power in medicine, and government intervention.[6] Amid this, an emphasis on "accountability" emerged in the 1980s and 1990s, which, in medicine, often focused on being subject to rules established by health care administrations. Although many physicians argue that this places barriers between patients and practitioners, others consider that bureaucracy is being used as an "excuse" for failings in their profession.[7] Many believe that, in order to restore professional values and public confidence, a clearly defined "social contract" is necessary between medicine and society, or the restoration of a covenant of trust, which is generally understood as a solemn promise to serve society.[8] Yet for this to be realized or sustained, practitioners need to respond to current concerns and expectations of the public, as emphasized in Chapter 7. There is, too, a need to respond to social factors that impinge on health care, for public concerns cover not only practitioners' responsibilities to individual patients, but also social determinants of community health.

Issues over the nature of professionalism exist throughout all segments of health care. A recent review of complementary medicine in Britain points out that many modalities have, through self-regulation, undertaken a process of "professionalization." The authors, in describing the latter as "occupational change and formation through unification, standardization, and the acquisition of external legitimacy," note that professionalization strategies have enabled chiropractors, reflexologists, and homeopaths to claim expertise and legitimacy, but concludes that, although "the groups of complementary practitioners we have studied have fully adopted the 'traits' of a profession which may bring greater legitimacy and preserve their practice . . . they have not secured the traditional rewards of autonomy and authority."[9]

The "traits" of the professions referred to in this quote are drawn from the writings of sociologists. For instance,

1. unification with agreement on the identity of the practice;
2. codification of knowledge through specialized education and core curricula;
3. self-regulation and social closure through limiting the number of practitioners and the establishment of strict training programs; and
4. alignment to the scientific paradigm.

What has not been acquired, say the authors, is another trait, namely social standing through support from strategic elites such as the state and powerful pressure groups. In fact, to attain this, as we indicated earlier, we believe that the group through its individual members must respond to public concerns and broad social issues that affect health.

Certainly, for public acceptance, there has to be much more than the commonly heard, superficial views that being a professional (not necessarily in health care) is "to be licensed and to follow a code of ethics," or being a highly skilled "knowledge worker" (i.e., merely a provider of expert services).[10] One is reminded of a Dilbert cartoon strip (by Scott Adams) that targets current glibness toward professionalism:

> "Anyone who takes more than thirty minutes for lunch is unprofessional."
> "That's still too long! I say you're unprofessional after six minutes."

"That's a little too professional, Wally."
"Death to those who eat!"[11]

Physicians and other health care practitioners are often unfamiliar with sociologist's views on professionalism, at least those that commonly focus attention on professional power and how it is acquired and sustained. Physicians, in contrast, commonly identify professionalism with such values as compassion, integrity, and humility, as well as upholding codes of ethics. Yet there are others who do not find it easy to define professionalism, for they see it as having an elusive, almost indefinable, quality. Recently, physician-author Michael LaCombe has said, "Professionalism is something everyone else seems to have more of than you yourself could ever hope for." It is, he says, a "matter of *being*"[12] For some, this is the same as saying that true professionalism comes from "within oneself." In other words, the characteristics of an individual contribute much to notions of professionalism. Personal values are important and, in ideal circumstances, are compatible with professional values.

In responding to the question, Who is a professional?, we believe that the different interpretations and views of sociologists, health care practitioners, patients, and also historians are relevant. The latter make clear, for instance, that professions have been characterized differently over time and place.[13] For example, in the early nineteenth century the English barrister was indubitably a member of a profession, yet the bar lacked any formal requirements for professional training and had no professional association.[14] Early modern physicians, too, commonly linked professionalism with being a gentlemen and a scholar, characteristics which are not seen in the same way in today's world of technological medicine.[15]

However one approaches being a professional, few would disagree that one aspect is the authority and power that sociologists' commonly see as a central aspect of professionalism. Disagreement may well exist about the extent of power and authority, for many factors are at play as we now consider.

AUTHORITY AND POWER

In recent decades, just as various social forces have been eroding the high social prestige, authority and power acquired by physicians in the "golden age" of medicine (the first half of the twentieth century), many commentators have been critical of misuse and abuses by physicians of their expertise and power.[16] Abuses are particularly prevalent, it has been said, when a profession is threatened by loss of authority, perhaps in uncertain times.[17] Misuse of power can be obvious or subtle. Sexual abuse contrasts sharply with the more subjective area of paternalism (the doctor "knows best" syndrome) which, nowadays is viewed as generally inappropriate because of respect for the autonomy and rights of patients. Yet many practitioners slide into inappropriate paternalism, especially when communication between practitioner and patient is not easy. What may be termed mild or soft paternalism is reflected in such comments as "This is what *I* would do," with the implication "You *ought* to do the same." This contrasts with emphatic paternalism, such as "This *must* be done" with no options being given.[18] Although little disquiet with the power of complementary/alternative practitioners has been expressed publicly, it does exist, including among skeptical family members of a patient, especially where there are no regulatory controls. Such concerns mean that all practitioners need to be aware of their authority and power and to recognize its imbalance in numerous practitioner-patient relationships.

A useful approach to considering the nature of any practitioner's power is Howard Brody's *The Healer's Power* (1992).[19] Brody describes three forms of doctors' power:

1. Aesculapian power that rests on specialized knowledge and skills and the privileges, accorded by society, such that practitioners are allowed to investigate intimately the body in health, illness, and death
2. Charismatic power reflecting a practitioner's personality
3. Social power arising from status and roles in society

Brody argues that the nature of power and its implications must be recognized in all areas of medical practice as a core issue in medical ethics. For instance, we have already questioned the directive of the Alberta College of Physicians and Surgeons that patients wait seventy-two hours before starting complementary/alternative treatment with a licensed physician. In another arena, some homeopaths are said to act paternalistically by not divulging their prescriptions to patients, for fear of misunderstandings over dilutions.

As helpful as Brody's approach is, we still need to recognize that his three forms of power are compounded from many factors. We review some of these in order to consider how a feeling of *belonging* to, rather than just being a member of a profession is fostered.

Professional Education and Knowledge

One key factor behind a sense of belonging to a profession is "cultural bonding," much of which depends on acquiring the profession's specialist knowledge as well as special titles (e.g., physician).[20] By specialist knowledge we mean more than, say, facts about a disease or understanding the "special" language of traditional Chinese medical theory. It also covers what is often called "clinical judgment." This is as much an issue in complementary/alternative as conventional care, if not more so.

Clinical Judgment and the Art and Tradition of Medicine

Clinical judgment, sometimes viewed as "tacit knowledge," is not easy to define, albeit readily recognized by experienced practitioners.[21] It is more than a systematic evaluation of data as taught in textbooks. Some see it as an almost intuitive ability in diagnosis, an ability—developed from experience—to identify critical signs or symptoms in a patient, amid much other, often confusing, data. In other words, a practitioner with good clinical judgment is able to separate wheat from chaff, perhaps in "reading" signs and symptoms, especially the more subjective ones such as "flattening of effect," and "severity of pain."[22]

Although clinical judgment has been described as the "art of medicine," the latter generally means more than astute diagnoses. It also refers to an ability to make humane judgments. This ability, too, relates to experience, but it can also be fostered by exploring the human condition through the humanities.[23] Certainly, knowledge of the history of a profession, its experiences in dealing with countless diseases, can contribute to clinical judgment, just as it can foster a sense of roots, of belonging. In this, oaths and codes can be significant. For instance, the Hippocratic oath and its modern versions—along with current discussions on making it pan-professional for all health professions—contributes as much to a sense of tradition as to a manifesto for current medical practice. This sense of tradition, felt keenly by many practitioners in conventional health professions, also owes much to a long history of the "greats": for example, great doctors, great professional institutions (lined with countless portraits of presidents and other medical celebrities), and great researchers. In emphasizing the "authorities" of the past, such celebratory history helps to validate the lineage of expert knowledge that contributes to defining a profession.

It is less clear whether students of complementary/alternative medicine are exposed to a similar sense of tradition, even though traditional Chinese, herbal, and homeopathic medicine, for example, stress a long history and the influence of great practitioners (e.g., Samuel Hahnemann as the founder of homeopathy). Moreover, Hippocrates is often seen as much a father of "natural" as conventional medicine. Yet, perhaps what is important for complementary/alternative medicine is not so much the celebratory history of the greats, but the need to understand the tradition of *opposition* to it and the problems of fragmentation through multiple organizations and educational institutions. Such fragmentation contrasts with medicine's key and powerful institutions, such as the American, British, and Canadian Medical Associations. Generally housed in striking and imposing buildings, they, like medical schools, boast a "solid" history of public service in part by promoting professional standards, education, medical advancement, and collegiality. As such they are not only part of a strong sense of tradition and belonging, but also do much to sustain it.

Institutions

Any exploration of the roots and traditions of medical institutions begins, as with so many other aspects of Western medicine, in ancient Greece. Conventional and complementary/alternative medicine (at least such concepts as working with the healing power of nature) trace their origins back to the time of Hippocrates (c. 450-370 B.M.E.). Then certain practitioners tried to establish "professional" boundaries to distinguish themselves from others who were perhaps recognized as quacks (to use modern terminology). However, the institutionalization of Western medicine, along with an acquisition of professional authority, only emerged between the eleventh and sixteenth centuries. Numerous factors played a part. One was the establishment of medicine as a separate faculty (like theology and law) in various universities of medieval Europe and Britain. Historians consider that medicine, by becoming part of higher learning, was able to "institutionalize" or to codify knowledge—to define what was orthodox knowledge and to set aside, "to marginalize," the unorthodox. The establishment of boundaries around orthodox care was further consolidated by the foundation of numerous associations of physicians that acquired local or regional authority to control the practice of medicine. By Renaissance times, such trends embraced an unwritten social "contract" between society and the medical profession which included protecting the public from "quackery," legacies of which persist.

It is clear that by early modern times medical authority and power owed much to its institutions. As already noted, critics have charged that this authority and power has not always been used responsibly. Certainly the attitudes of medical organizations are not always easy to interpret, even with hindsight, as to whether activities are genuine efforts to serve society or whether they are more self-serving. After all, many people have difficulty over understanding, as anything but self-serving, the twentieth-century efforts by the American Medical Association to prevent universal health insurance in the United States.

Another episode, an earlier one, that also serves as an interesting example of professional values being seemingly out of step with social responsibilities merits mention, if only because it also helped to precipitate a shift in professional roles. The Royal College of Physicians of London, in the seventeenth century, despite a rapidly growing population in London as well as countless social problems precipitated by a civil war and outbreaks of plague, maintained a stable number of physician fellows of the College—fewer than forty for most of the century. In so doing, it failed to respond to the needs of an expanding population. Although this may be seen as exhibiting professional power in times of stress for the College, it ultimately contributed to the emergence—from the ranks of apothecaries—of other medical practitioners with no allegiance to the Royal College.[24]

This episode of shifting professional roles invites comparisons with trends today and the likely emergence of new divisions of labor in health care. Greater participation in diagnosis and therapy from, say, nurses, nurse practitioners, physician assistants, and pharmacists was already underway by 2000, just as numerous complementary/alternative practitioners established themselves, in health care. Unquestionably, all health organizations and educational institutions need to continually reevaluate the changing health care and sociocultural scene. Is it possible that "belonging" to a particular health profession may take on a sense of belonging to *the* health profession, rather than to a particular branch?

Hospitals and the Institutionalization of Medicine

Any consideration of medicine's sources of authority and power, of the sense of belonging among practitioners, must notice the complex role hospitals play.

> The hospital is in some ways peculiarly characteristic of our society. Within the walls of a single building, high technology, bureaucracy, and professionalism are juxtaposed with the most fundamental and unchanging human experiences—birth, death, pain. It is no accident that black comedy and soap opera should have found the hospital a natural setting. It is an institution clothed with an almost mystical power, yet suffused with a relentless impersonality and a forbidding aura of technical complexity.[25]

Although the story of hospitals extends back to the Middle Ages and earlier, the expression "hospital medicine" only emerges—in the sense of it being a specialty—in the twentieth century. Even so, the role of hospitals as a fountainhead of medicine and research, rather than solely a place to care for and treat the sick, had arisen earlier. During the eighteenth century, for instance, hospitals—then increasing in numbers and hence bringing more patients together with similar conditions—emerged as "resources" for physicians and students to study "diseases."

Subsequently during the nineteenth and first half of the twentieth century hospitals became centers of medical education, research, and scientific medicine. In the 1800s they fostered the development of the then relatively new clinico-pathological approach to medicine. This was the "search for a lesion," in other words, correlating signs and symptoms with specific pathology in organs, tissues, or body fluids. By defining the basis of medical practice in this way, it came, as we noted earlier, to be vigorously opposed to "nonscientific" alternative practices such as homeopathy.[26] The twentieth-century hospital story is primarily one of expansion and new roles as repositories of complex technology for diagnosis and therapy, all of which added to the growth of medicine's authority and to an emphasis on effective institutional functioning not always compatible with sensitive total care of patients. As has been said, by 1920 the hospital was an institution that became "medicalized" while the medical profession itself became "hospitalized."

The story of the hospital impinges on that of complementary/alternative medicine in many ways. Noteworthy is the virtual demise in the early decades of the twentieth century of, for instance, various homeopathic hospitals and of other institutions (often called sanatoria) for alternative treatment (some for drug and alcohol addiction, nervousness, etc.). In terms of the current professional standing of complementary/alternative medicine, the demise of the hospital has been particularly unfortunate. Whether some of the authority that goes with hospital care will be recovered as complementary/alternative therapy is introduced into hospitals remains to be seen. Certainly pressures exist to integrate complementary/alternative care within hospitals, with calls to do away with rules that prohibit the use of alternative medicine. "The change would leave patients and doctors free to make conscientious decisions about a treatment."[27]

The Office and Other Symbols of Authority

Although hospitals have a key role in underpinning the authority of medical and allied health professionals, practitioners' offices also deserve consideration. Do they serve to contribute to the authority of a practitioner? Do they make a patient feel comfortable, and not be intimidated although in a doctor's space? Are they conducive to positive therapeutic outcomes? Does an office within a "fancy" clinic or a shopping center make a difference? Should practitioners consider the concept of "therapeutic landscapes," or how particular locations and settings are associated with healing or contribute to holistic care.[28] Although there are no general answers to these questions, if only because patients differ in what makes them feel comfortable, few doubt that offices and their setting—as well as such other symbols of medical practice as stethoscopes and white coats—can be significant in creating professional identity and contributing to therapeutic outcomes.[29] Certainly the impact of offices on patients has long been recognized.[30] Recently, in 1991, Anatole Broyard wrote convincingly as a patient sitting in a doctor's office:

> I read [the physician's] signs. The diplomas I took for granted. What interested me was the fact that the room was furnished with taste. There were well-made, well-filled bookcases, an antique desk and chairs, a reasonable Oriental rug on the floor. . . . On the walls and desk were pictures of three healthy-looking conspicuously happy children, photographed in a prosperous

outdoor setting of lawn, flowers and trees. As I remember, one of the photographs showed a sailboat. From the evidence, their father knew how to live—and, by extension, how to look after the lives of others. His magic seemed good.[31]

Although not everyone would feel comfortable in such elegance and money (they may see it as ostentatious), handsome offices with handsome furniture have always had a "message" of success and stability. Likewise, although less so recently, sartorial elegance was part of the image of success. Much has been written on the appropriate appearance of physicians, and caricaturists have consistently called on dress and appearance to document public attitudes to the profession.[32] For instance, until around the 1950s, doctors were commonly caricatured as elegantly dressed, often in tails and pinstripe trousers. By then, however, the white coat had become a widely recognized symbol; in symbolizing medical science more than patient care, the white coat is also to be seen as a mask that hides the real person.[33] There are clearly reasons why some physicians shun white coats, almost preferring the image of an avuncular country doctor that is so much a part of the romantic imagery of medicine of the past.[34] All this is as much an issue for complementary/alternative practitioners who wish to present the concept of holistic care.

Countless practitioners have always said that the "trappings" of success were unimportant compared with quality care, though making patients feel comfortable and not intimidated can itself contribute to this. To some extent this is reflected in waiting room design that pays attention to, for example, ready accessibility for the disabled and to infection control. Many complementary/alternative practitioners stress that paying attention to details—from offering water or tea to patients to the absence of judgmental waiting room literature on public health matters—adds to the therapeutic environment. Further, hanging family photographs on the wall may be inappropriate in many practices, although they might deserve consideration in the office as a way of providing a human touch to the persona of the practitioner.

Gender and Professional Images

A quip attributed to celebrated physician Sir William Osler (1849-1919) goes, "There are three classes of human beings: men, women and women physicians." Nowadays, any consideration of professional images and authority must consider the impact of women practitioners and the changes they bring. Osler, of course, lived at a time when medicine was a male profession with few women physicians. Although this is no longer the case, with dramatic increases in the number of women entering medicine in recent years, there are those who still consider that medicine—especially surgery—continues to be dominated by male values, which are commonly seen as placing less concern on caring, nurturing, and empathy than do women (see also Modern Bioethics, in this chapter). Legacies of gender bias are evident at times such as the 1999 controversy over a Thai beauty queen, a psychiatrist. The male-dominated psychiatry establishment stated, "a beauty queen cannot be a good psychiatrist, since patients can relate to her in an inappropriate way."[35] Behind such image issues also lies the implication that females possess less technical ability than men.[36]

Such matters have not generally arisen in complementary/alternative medicine. In fact, the field as a whole has been described as "female," not so much on the basis of gender composition of practitioners, but because its emphasis on holism is considered to fit feminine values of caring and nurturing. It is argued that it empowers women to take control of their health.[37] All this seems to draw upon a long history of "wise" women, and women healers, and the way society associates gentleness, empathy, and nurturance with women. Of course, just as many men have these characteristics, and not all women practitioners portray them. Women—and it cannot be said that all demonstrate such characteristics—need to consider whether the expectations patients have of them are different from expectations of male practitioners.

OATHS AND CODES

Introduction

Any consideration of authority and power raises questions about whether practitioners themselves recognize their power. Are they able to monitor how the power is used? We ask here about the role of oaths and codes. Do they play a significant part in professional behavior, or are they mostly window dressing?

Despite the longevity of the Hippocratic oath (see below), codes of ethics only became a conspicuous aspect of medical professionalism in the nineteenth century. It can be argued that only now are we in the heyday of health care codes with the late twentieth-century emergence of many new ones including from complementary/alternative medicine.[38] In part because of the plethora of new codes, a single ethical code or oath for every practitioner in health care, a panprofessional oath, has been proposed, one deserving of attention by complementary/alternative medicine groups.[39] However, as in the past, doubts continue about the value of oaths and codes. Do many practitioners remember their contents except in the most general of ways? Many view them, as has long been the case, as much less important than the character of a practitioner.[40] On the other hand, oaths are increasingly considered to indicate more than professional behavior. Oaths are statements of standards, certainly more than window dressing. We include the British General Medical Council's 1998 succinct statement on "duties," (see Box 6.1) with the implication of a binding mandate as a noteworthy response to new public concerns. The focus is only on patients, hence it is limited in scope, but it prompts reflection on the responsibilities or duties of all practitioners.

BOX 6.1. A Physician's Duties

General Medical Council in Britain

If, in the past, a somewhat informal approach was taken toward codes of ethics in Britain, the General Medical Council now makes clear the importance of standards. The following statement (1998) has been circulated by the Council to all physicians on the British register. (See text.)

The duties of a doctor registered with the General Medical Council.

Patients must be able to trust doctors with their lives and well-being. To justify that trust, we as a profession have a duty to maintain a good standard of practice and care and to show respect for human life. In particular as a doctor you must:

- make the care of your patient your first concern;
- treat every patient politely and considerately;
- respect patients' dignity and privacy;
- listen to patients and respect their views;
- give patients information in a way they can understand;
- respect the rights of patients to be fully involved in decisions about their care;
- keep your professional knowledge and skills up to date;
- recognize the limits of your professional competence;
- be honest and trustworthy;
- respect and protect confidential information;

(continued)

(continued)

- make sure that your personal beliefs do not prejudice your patients' care;
- act quickly to protect patients from risk if you have good reason to believe that you or a colleague may not be fit to practise;
- avoid abusing your position as a doctor; and
- work with colleagues in the ways that best serve patients' interests.

In all these matters you must never discriminate unfairly against your patients or colleagues. And you must always be prepared to justify your actions to them.

The question of what material to include in oaths and codes always arouses much debate. For instance, to what extent should they be limited to basic principles and values, and what specific prohibitions should be included? Nevertheless, few would disagree that in evaluating oaths and codes, at least the following, somewhat overlapping, points need consideration. Do they:

1. Make clear the moral values that the profession sees as fundamentally important for professional responsibilities?
2. Indicate practice standards not only for the guidance of practitioners, but also for the information of patients and of society in general?
3. Address professional power and recognize its potential abuse?
4. Contribute to professional coherence and tradition by defining the boundaries of professional practice, and indicate the responsibilities of the individual practitioner?
5. Demonstrate responsiveness to current social needs and concerns?

As all organizations—conventional and complementary/alternative—constantly evaluate such considerations, they also need to consider whether an ethical code should be developed as a clear social contract with society, either as a covenant, in the sense of a public pledge to serve society, or as a written contract negotiated with society.

The Hippocratic Oath

Although the most celebrated of all oaths, the Hippocratic oath (written around 400 B.M.E.), is generally associated with mainstream medicine, some complementary/alternative practitioners make clear they work within the Hippocratic tradition, in part because of a Hippocratic emphasis on diet. Certainly, its tradition merits consideration by all health care practitioners. Indeed, one of the panprofessional oaths that has been proposed is a modernized Hippocratic oath.

The early history of the oath and different interpretations about its purpose in classical times have prompted much debate. However, this is more of academic interest than of current professional interest because the oath has been constantly modified over the centuries to fit changing mores. Certainly, until it was adapted in the Middle Ages to Christian, Muslim, and Jewish faiths, the oath had little influence. Thereafter it developed into a veritable medical "tradition," although more one of spirit than detail. The prohibitions in the original oath—that ban surgery by physicians, use of a deadly drug, even if asked for, and abortions—cannot have the same meanings today. It is more the essence of the oath that attracts interest, commonly interpreted as a practitioner's first obligation being to the individual patient. In fact, some see it as patient-centered care, which can be paternalistic (as is the oath in places) and hence inappropriate for practice today. [41]

The Hippocratic oath is by no means the only ethical challenge to the interpretative skills of historians, partly because the social circumstances in which oaths and codes were initially developed have changed. The often discussed 1803 book, *Medical Ethics; or, a Code of Institutes and Precepts Adapted to the Professional Conduct of Physicians and Surgeons* by Thomas Percival in England has prompted various opinions about its significance. Precipitated in part by disputes among physicians and surgeons in new hospitals, the book offered practical suggestions that influenced many later codes. It reflects Percival's concerns that declining professional and personal standards in the last decades of the eighteenth century—encouraged by ambition, career-mindedness, and personal glory—jeopardized humanism.[42] *Medical Ethics* gives us the eighteenth-century meaning of a "good" physician. Although this notion was being affected by a changing medical world (e.g., the growing number of hospitals, and various efforts to make medicine more open or understandable to the public), for most people the good physician remained one who possessed gentlemanly and Christian manners and virtues that mirrored the moral and humanistic ideals of the eighteenth-century Enlightenment.[43]

Of particular interest is the influence of Percival's *Medical Ethics* in North America where it contributed much to the formalizing and codifying of medical ethics. Inadvertently, perhaps, this fostered a view that professionalism had as much to do with observing a code of ethics as with innate virtuous behavior. Although different interpretations of Percival's influence exist, the American Medical Association code of 1847 drew on his *Medical Ethics* in outlining what might be seen as a social contract between the profession and society. The introduction to the Association's first code stated:

> Every duty or obligation implies, both in equity and for its successful discharge, a corresponding right. As it is the duty of a physician . . . to expose his health and life for the benefit of the community, he has a just claim in return on all its members, collectively and individually.[44]

However, society in general hardly had input into the nature of the code. Moreover, it is far from certain that all physicians construed the code as in any way a contract with society. Perhaps they saw Percival and the AMA code as primarily a guidance to medical etiquette at a time of many inter- and intraprofessional squabbles, though not all commentators agree. It must be said that professional etiquette tends to get relatively little formal attention today in our climate of patient-centered care, though it is an important issue, especially at a time when efforts are being made to develop team care (see Chapter 7). Nor is much attention given to the sense of honor in being a member of a group? While this matter has only been studied in the context of the professions in North America, it is an issue for physicians and other health care practitioners on both sides of the Atlantic.[45] As much as anything it has raised and raises questions about honorable behavior with colleagues.

Codes of ethics, as they are "revised," reflect their times. For instance, nowadays there is a clear sense that current concerns with autonomy and patients' rights must be considered as part of any code. Amid the many ethical concerns and emphasis on accountability that mark the beginning of the 2000s, there are calls, at least in North America, for more explicit statements about the ethical principles on which a code is based rather than leaving them as "do's" and "don'ts." Making clear the principles on which a code is based, not only helps a professional body to justify codes as standards, but also prompts consideration of the relationship between personal and professional values. As we have noted, a compatibility between such values is per-haps necessary for an individual's feeling of being a professional.

Given changes in codes over time, as well as national differ-ences—for instance, compared to the U.S., the British medical pro-fession has not had a formal code as such—it can be constructive to study the history of codes to get a sense of changing views on recur-ring issues. For instance, eighteenth-century attitudes toward the compatibility of medicine and business contrasted sharply with later views that point up constant professional-commercial tensions.[46]

Complementary/Alternative Medicine Codes

Our discussion so far emphasizes that oaths and codes are an impor-tant part of a profession's identity. Complementary/alternative medi-cine organizations commonly give priority to formulating codes, of which a great diversity now exist. Moreover, at least some organiza-tions demand that new members must follow conventional medical oaths.[47] A useful discussion by Julie Stone and Joan Matthews high-light some general issues. First, they express concerns (as we have done) over the failure of new codes to make clear the principles on which they are based:

> [Codes] rarely adumbrate the full range of ethical principles which practitioners need to be aware of. Concepts such as truth-fulness, which give rise to intense discussion within health care, are rarely dealt with. Nor do codes tend to question justice is-sues, such as access to grievance procedures and compensation for harm.[48]

A principal difficulty with codes is that they tend to be designed by professionals for professionals. "As such, they face the criticism that is most frequently leveled against self-regulating bodies, namely that they are not independent and do not involve the consumer."[49]

Stone and Matthews illustrate the diversity of existing codes by contrasting those of the British Complementary Medical Association (BCMA) and the Institute of Complementary Medicine (ICM), also in the United Kingdom. Aside from internal inconsistencies in the codes, overall they reveal significant differences over interactions be-tween complementary therapists and orthodox health care profes-sionals. The BCMA code makes clear that complementary therapists are to be seen as adjunct to or complementary to orthodox medicine:

"the registered medical practitioner must remain in charge of the patient's treatment and clinically accountable for the care offered by the complementary therapist." In emphasizing this, the BCMA code insists that complementary practitioners may *not* make a "medical diagnosis," a directive considered to protect the practitioner from potential legal liability. However, Stone and Matthews point out that this is at variance "with what practitioners routinely do and need to do in order to treat a patient."[50]

The Institute of Complementary Medicine (ICM) code contrasts significantly with that of the BCMA on the matter of diagnosis. Although the patient may bring to a consultation a medical history based on allopathic diagnoses, the code recognizes that "every practitioner irrespective of status or technique must make an initial medical diagnostic assessment of the condition of the patient/client and note the result on a record card."[51] However, it goes on to state that "no attempt should be made to describe a complementary diagnosis in allopathic terms unless the practitioner is so qualified."

Such differences between codes prompt specific questions for organizations. For example, to what extent do complementary/alternative codes balance (1) serving the profession by defining practitioners' responsibilities to the group and (2) serving the best interests of patients, including respect for their autonomy? To what extent do the codes open the door to conflict between personal moral values and professional values (e.g., advice over abortion). And, how helpful are codes that are largely a shopping list of do's and dont's, a mix of values and professional directives? For instance, the code of The American Herbalists Guild addresses the following in bullet form: Honesty, Confidentiality, Professional Courtesy, Professional Networking, Practitioner as Educator, Peer Review, Referring Out, Avoiding Needless Therapy, Environment Commitment, and Sexual Harassment.[52] All are important issues, but as a potpourri of points, they are devoid of stated principles and context, and thereby, not easy to remember.

MODERN BIOETHICS

Introduction

We have noted that Stone and Matthews promote "ethics-led" regulation (see discussion on regulation in Chapter 5). They are clearly influenced by modern bioethics, which in covering, for example, the ethics of reproductive technologies and of social policies, is broader in scope than traditional medical ethics. Bioethics also has a more public face and, as a social movement like complementary/alternative medicine, it became increasingly prominent from the 1960s onward, although bioethics emerged more from academic rather than grass roots.

Bioethics identified itself in the 1960s as a result of various concerns that added to the Nazi atrocities committed in the name of eugenic "science" during World War II. There were exposés, from both sides of the Atlantic, of questionable research ethics. In Britain, physician Maurice Pappworth's "Human Guinea Pigs—A Warning" (1962) was a first volley in his extended campaign to raise public debate.[53] This, with an analogous article by Henry Beecher in the United States (1966), contributed to making "invisible issues visible," in other words, bringing ethical problems in research and, by extension, in clinical practice out into the open.[54]

This new public visibility was also related to and fostered by interrelated factors such as technological changes, sociopolitical unrest, and activism that encouraged critical examination of health care, of practitioners, and of the rights of patients. The 1962 tragedy of iatrogenic birth defects from a new drug, thalidomide, galvanized further bioethical questions. Furthermore, trends toward the use of more and more expensive medical technology not only fostered additional concerns about whether medicine was being dehumanized, but also highlighted scarce financial resources for health care. For instance, in the 1960s lay decision making in Seattle, Washington, attracted much debate and scrutiny regarding who could and could not be dialyzed.[55] From this time on, an increasingly better informed public—in part due to consumerism, feminism, civil liberties, human rights, media coverage, film and TV scripts, and multiculturalism—contributed to a widening of interest in bioethics. In the 1970s, the celebrated case of Karen Ann Quinlan (successful court arguments, 1975-1976, to turn off her life support technology) was a watershed that indicated physicians were no longer the sole authority in matters of ethics. Indeed, medical ethics had become subsumed under bioethics.[56]

During the emergence of bioethics, philosophers brought forward various moral theories for analyzing ethical dilemmas in health care, at a time when, it is said, physicians began to call upon ethicists in the hope of shifting the burden for difficult decisions. A large body of specialist literature now exists, and we offer some parallel reading to this volume.[57] Although philosophical medical ethics has been the main feature of bioethics' development, concerns exist that the views of philosopher/ethicists can differ substantially from those of practitioners whose own experiences (see discussion of casuistry) shape ethical decision making. However, that is not to say that principles of philosophical bioethics are not supported in everyday practice through religious and cultural factors. We comment first, in the following notes, on principlism, which has had a marked impact on health care in general, before looking at other approaches to ethical dilemmas.

Principlism

The philosophical approach that has attracted the greatest attention is principlism. Four principles (autonomy, beneficence, nonmaleficence, and justice) have become especially well known in North America and elsewhere through the writings of T. L. Beauchamp and J. F. Childress.[58] First, we should ask do we need "principles"? Our contemporary world is highly pluralistic, not only through ethnic, cultural, and religious diversity, but also through different understandings of moral values. Thus it is not surprising that many people are inclined to see ethics generally as a private matter such that each individual determines his or her own ethical values. Societal and interpersonal relationships, however, limit this privacy. Without some agreement, life and social relationships would be impossible. Agreement commonly rests on some sense of generalizability, or universality—a defining characteristic of a principle. In other words, a principle will apply to many and not just to single cases. For example, it would be unethical, because of extensive experience with countless cases of diabetes, to *treat* a patient with the disease without offering them education in how they should look after themselves to lessen the risk of complications.

Clearly, then, principles are a core aspect of moral theory. An ethical analysis based on principles is often described as the epitome of "top down" (also known as duty-based or deontological) ethics. This means that principles are applied to analyze an ethical case on moral grounds irrespective of special circumstances and the consequences. However, in specifically commenting on the principlism commonly employed in bioethical analysis, and on some relevant issues arising from complementary/alternative medicine, we note first that the approach is not solely top-down since beneficence and nonmaleficence are generally evaluated in the context of the particular circumstances of the case.

The Principle of Autonomy

Ethicists are not alone in agreeing that the minimal requirement of any ethically good relationship is mutual respect for the other person, in other words, respect for the autonomy of the person and the recognition of his or her right to make decisions. Any practitioner, therefore, who infringes on the rights of patients to decide on matters affecting their own well-being would, at least prima facie, disregard this principle. Ensuring informed consent, personal freedom of the patient, patients' rights, truth-telling, confidentiality, and sharing decision making, all hinge on this general principle.

A general class of infringements would be those which reflect what has come to be called the "old" paternalism of physicians ("doctors know best") that we have already raised. If, for various reasons, the patient is not competent to make decisions (e.g., due to being a minor, or due to mental incompetence), a decision on the part of a practitioner to override autonomy is not necessarily immoral; however, the point of the principle is that the presumption must always be in favor of autonomy, even where children and mentally ill patients are concerned.

Autonomy is often an unacknowledged issue in complementary/alternative care. For instance, is it commonly overlooked when physicians fail to respect a patient's wish for their help with complementary/alternative medicine? In contrast, pharmacists who sell natural health products, but allow customers to choose from an array of products often argue that they are respecting customers' autonomy. However, this approach of "buyer beware" may well not fulfil professional responsibility "to do no harm."

The Principle of Beneficence

Although this is widely interpreted as practitioners doing what is best for patients, debate exists about the precise meaning of the term. It can be viewed as a prerequisite for a practitioner-patient relationship, for it can reasonably be assumed that the patient goes to a practitioner for health reasons and that the practitioner is expected to be both knowledgeable and capable. Consequently, what is implicit in a beneficent relationship between them is that the practitioner will provide the best possible medical service and quality of care.

However, doing what is best for a patient is not always as straightforward as many would like to believe. The uncertainty of medicine can make it difficult to decide on the best treatment for, say, arthritis, and even to improve the quality of life of sufferers. There are many dilemmas. For instance, although complementary/alternative practitioners commonly assess improvement in "wellness" on the basis of a patient's self-assessment, objective (e.g., blood) tests may suggest the basic problem is unchanged. This prompts the question: To what extent should complementary/alternative practitioners evaluate the nature of scientific evidence as part of their responsibility in doing what is best for patients?

The Principle of Nonmaleficence

In some ways this principle, namely the long-standing medical aphorism, "to do no harm," appears to be simply the flip-side of beneficence. While uncertainty is often expressed over the real difference between beneficence and non-maleficence, the latter does signal a particular emphasis. It reminds the practitioner of the need to assess risks, and to evaluate risks versus benefits.

Although nonmaleficence is generally seen as an issue for mainstream medicine, it is just as important for complementary/alternative practice with all the public concerns over safety and lack of standards that we raised earlier. This goes beyond specific safety issues to such matters as avoiding financial exploitation of patients by, for instance, high fees or recommending unnecessary preparations. There is, too, the contentious issue of making a diagnosis that is viewed as idiosyncratic, at least by mainstream practitioners. For instance, in Part III (case history/reading 8) we raise the issue of diagnosing allergies without administering specific challenges of the allergen to a patient.

Nonmaleficence, too, raises questions about the responsibility of a practitioner to foresee (and to act accordingly on) various social and environmental problems that can negatively affect a person's health. (See discussion on health advocacy.)

The Principle of Justice

In traditional Christian ethics a distinction was often made between justice and charity. The former covers all matters which could be considered as absolute duty; the latter extends beneficence to more positively benevolent or loving actions, something beyond the range and scope of obligation. In the context of contemporary medical ethics, questions about justice commonly arise in the context of extending considerations from the individual to collective interests, perhaps to counteract what some see as excessive individualism in medicine, or an excessive emphasis on autonomy. The norms or requirements of this principle in health care can be stated as: "Other things being equal, all patients have an equal right to good and effective treatment for their health problems." Implementing this, however, opens the proverbial "can of worms" of social and political issues. For instance, political parties everywhere have their differences of opinion as to what constitutes fairness. Does it mean equal access or only to whatever one can afford? Hotly debated issues in Canada and the United Kingdom are "two-tier" and "user-pay" systems (as exists in the United States) versus universal coverage by the state, both of which raise issues about the meaning of justice in health care.

Issues over interpretation of justice permeate the health care of individuals in many other ways. For example, while confidentiality is recognized as central to the physician-patient relationship, circumstances exist in which strict observance of a patient's confidentiality constitutes a threat to the rights of a third party to information necessary for his or her well-being. An example is whether to respect the confidentiality of a patient who is diagnosed as HIV positive and who wishes this to be concealed from his or her sexual partner. The decision must take into account any relevant public health legislation that mandates disclosure.

If, as is sometimes said, the principle of justice in bioethics raises more questions than it solves, it does bring important issues into sharp focus. For the complementary/alternative medicine practitioner, justice is an everyday issue where, for example, insurance coverage is limited, unavailable or inadequate, and where national health schemes offer no coverage. In this context, it is noteworthy that some support groups for users of complementary/alternative medicine develop funds for those who cannot afford its high cost. The extent to which activism is needed to bring about social justice is for the consideration of everyone.

Some Concerns

It is important to appreciate that concerns exist over the preoccupation with the four principles, especially autonomy. One reason is the need to deal with many situations when two principles clash; for instance, when practitioners feel they must respect a patient's decisions about health care (i.e., respect autonomy), while knowing such decisions may harm the patient (thus violating the principle of non-maleficence or to do no harm).

Another concern over the current emphasis on principlism is that, in characterizing so much of bioethics in the United States, it is shaped by the individualism of American culture. As a result, its relevance to health care in other cultures—despite our increasingly globalized medicine—is questioned. Indeed, the emphasis on the four principles has been criticized by European scholars who have suggested that a focus should be more on such concepts as liberty, therapeutic wholeness, and social subsidiarity, and on an understanding of nature, human community, and the human condition.[59]

Other Approaches to Ethical Dilemmas

Although students, on first learning about the variety of ethical teachings, tend to see ethics as a matter of opinion—a form of moral relativism—the different perspectives have a practical value. They serve as reminders of the many different factors to be considered in making moral decisions and different weightings that are given to them. They serve, too, to help individuals to consider whether, by nature or temperament, they lean toward the "top-down" approach (application of principles regardless of consequences), or to "bottom-up" and other ethical positions noted next.

"Bottom-Up" Ethics: Consequentialism, Social Utilitarianism

"Bottom-up" ethical approaches consider specific situations and consequences. For instance, as indicated in considering the principles of beneficence and nonmaleficence, consequences must be assessed. In practice, this can mean assessing the goodness or badness of consequences, that is, assessing prognoses or outcomes both medically and socially such as an impact on relatives.

In one well-known form of consequentialism—utilitarianism—ethicists use the language of maximizing the overall utility in any situation. This is often applied in such as way that a utilitarian decision will result in the greatest good for the greatest number of people in a community. Very often the issue that emerges is whether a practitioner's greatest responsibility is to the individual (a traditional medical ethic) or to the community. For instance, does reporting a notifiable infectious disease undermine the confidentiality owed to a patient? A broader example is allocation of scarce financial resources, where money spent on, say, expensive transplant surgery may reduce the quality of care for others. Of closer concern to patients wanting complementary/alternative care is whether public funds should be available to them.

Virtue Ethics

There is little disagreement that the core of ethics that has long shaped medicine—indeed until well past the establishment of formal codes in the nineteenth century—was "virtue" ethics. Although the concept of virtue (or virtues) is often loosely defined, it focuses on *innate* characteristics (or pattern of characteristics) that underpin morally good behavior. Until relatively recently, it was held that being born into the role of a gentleman and a Christian brought with it the virtues that went with those positions. It is not without interest that English seventeenth- and eighteenth-century testimonials that supported the local licensing of physicians and surgeons by church bishops—and seemingly expressed public expectations of practitioners— spoke not only of skills in "physick and chirurgery," but also of such virtues as "honest behaviour," "man of sober life and conservation," and "a person of civill and honest behaviour."[60] Innate virtues, however, could (and were to) be strengthened by a humanistic education to create the "good" physician. In fact, a clear sense exists that certain characteristics (e.g., the ideal physician is a scholar) were promoted in, for example, the eighteenth century as one way to strengthen a sense of professional identity.[61]

There are those who feel that, in the face of the modern emphasis on principlism, insufficient interest exists today in virtue ethics. In fact we have noticed that a tendency emerged for them to be given less attention when codes of ethics became formalized in the nineteenth century. E. D. Pellegrino has tried to bring about a more balanced approach. While he makes clear that a place still exists for principles in ethical analysis, the issue concerns how principles are applied. Pellegrino suggests that the following virtues need to be part of every practitioner's character: truthfulness, benevolence, effacement of self-interest, compassion and caring, intellectual honesty, justice, and prudence.[62] Such virtues—no less than lists of values recognized and highlighted by medical organizations and physicians (compare Values in Health Care, in Chapter 3)—can, of course, underpin the particular *attitudes* that patients wish to see in their health care practitioners.

In summary, we consider that as a basis for ethical behavior virtues and appropriate attitudes can be both innate and acquired by learning of which the humanities are considered important for prompting self-reflection.

Feminist and Feminine or Caring Ethics: Women and Men's Health

Nowadays no ethical analysis can omit the possibility that gender issues may be relevant. After all, women's concerns have become increasingly conspicuous throughout society. Among general matters raised with regard to health care is whether mainstream and complementary/alternative women practitioners, as part of their professional responsibility, should support the efforts of feminists to eliminate societal attitudes that subordinate women in society. In fact some see at least certain complementary/alternative modalities (e.g., homeopathy) as challenging conventional medicine and its stances on gender. [63]

We cannot explore the many challenges from feminist writers and others, beyond noting a few points.[64]

1. Although women are most commonly involved in health care (e.g., looking after other family members such as children, elderly parents and disabled adults), most conventional physicians have been male. Although medical school enrollment is correcting the imbalance, the question remains whether this will really address women's demands for greater awareness of women's health with its own specialist literature and iconic texts such as *Our Bodies, Ourselves: A Book by and for Women from the Boston Women's Health Book Collective* (first issued 1969).[65] Are women's health issues being taught in medical schools, a question also to be asked of complementary/alternative medicine? (The question can be asked, too: Are professionals responding to growing lay interest in men's health?)[66]

2. Mainstream medicine has been slow to investigate the possibility of complementary/alternative treatment even in areas such as hormone replacement therapy, which causes much angst among women.

3. Society's approach to research and what is worthy of particular attention has been negatively influenced by gender. For instance, health conditions affecting women have been relatively ignored in the past. Historically, for instance, albeit recently changing, very little

funding has gone into breast cancer research, while cardiac disease was viewed predominantly as a man's problem, thus omitting women from clinical trials. Further, many drug trials have focused on men because of the presumption that a female's hormones and pregnancies might complicate results. Collective responsibilities exist among the health professions to redress such issues.

In contrast to femi*nist* ethics—concerned with making political changes and eliminating oppressive imbalances of power—femi*nine* ethics (or caring ethics as it is often called) has, as its primary concept, the moral experience and intuitions of women. This approach arose, in part, from widespread interest in Carol Gilligan's 1982 publication *In a Different Voice: Psychological Theory and Women's Development.*[67] Gilligan characterizes both distinct masculine and feminine voices in ethical reasoning, whereas, as generally held, such reasoning has been carried on in an overwhelmingly masculine voice.

Gilligan argues that women are more inclined to perceive moral dilemmas primarily in terms of personal attachment versus detachment. A female's moral universe tends to be a world of relationships and psychological truths in which an awareness of connections between people gives rise to a ready appreciation of responsibility for one another. This moral orientation, most prevalent among females, was dubbed by Gilligan "ethic of care."[68]

In contrast, Gilligan feels that the principal moral orientation of males tends to focus on concerns related to inequality versus equality of individuals. This approach emphasizes "abstract" ideals of fairness and rights, and requires abiding by such principles as justice. It is noteworthy that the ethics of care has become central to nursing theory. Indeed, the nursing profession has adopted it as its own basic ethic of nursing, somewhat distinct from medical ethics. This distinction, however, is problematic since it might be interpreted that physicians don't "care" (they only "cure") and that their patients need an advocate. Clearly, complementary/alternative medicine, as it deals with issues of professionalism, has an opportunity to face all these issues constructively.

Casuistry

Physicians widely recognize that, in evaluating ethical problems, they often call upon their experiences of similar situations. Clinical practice in general is very much based on a practitioner's experience of previous cases, and we believe this has also long been a factor in making ethical decisions. Such decision making, calling on experience, is known as casuistry. As a formal approach to making decisions, casuistry extends back to the medieval Jesuitical tradition in which decisions were made by comparison with previous "index" ("cardinal" or "paradigm") cases of undoubted importance. It has been said that "casuistry bridges the gap between the speculative doctrines of philosophy and theology and the practical demands of decision making in particular circumstances."[69]

Building up experiences of ethical issues by comparison and analogy does not mean, as is sometimes suggested, that ethical principles are not at play. Casuistry, through cases, calls on a variety of moral theories, although since outcomes are an integral part of any case history, consequentialism can be especially evident. Furthermore, as the formal teaching of philosophical ethics teaching currently penetrates the health care professions more deeply new problems for younger doctors are more likely to be shaped by such teaching. We might add, too, that in so far as some also see a close kinship between casuistry and the use of patient's narratives, the latter can be viewed as case histories that extend personal experiences.[70]

Some General Comments

Where do these discussions on ethical approaches and perspectives leave us? Some suggest, cynically, that ethical analysis and decisions often reflect biases associated with one's primary discipline (e.g., medicine, nursing, or philosophy). This viewpoint reinforces the importance of a key step in our systematic approach to an ethical issue, namely the need to understand one's own particular ethical approach (e.g., reliance on principles alone, influenced by feminist perspectives, or other considerations.) A recent textbook on ethics notices the role of autonomy, beneficence and justice in decision making and adds, "Are there other situational factors that are important? Consider your conscience and emotional reactions, the actions of your peers, institutional policies and guidelines, professional norms, and legal precedents."[71] It can be problematic when, in calling on various factors unsystematically, a practitioner may not be able to make clear his or her reasoning behind reaching a particular decision.[72]

It is worth stressing here that the moral framework of medical practice can change imperceptibly, as can one's own values. For instance, despite many initial concerns when organ transplants emerged, it soon became an accepted "treatment" so that organs have almost become commodities like drugs. There are issues, too, about acceding to patients' requests for certain treatments (e.g., antibiotics), while recognizing that doing so may not be in accord with professional values.

NOTES

1. For medicine as a "model" to study professions, see J. C. Burnham, "How the Idea of Profession Changed the Writing of Medical History," *Medical History,* Supplement No. 18, 1998.

2. B. Lown, *The Lost Art of Healing,* Boston: Houghton Miflin, 1996, p. xi. For professionalism in "peril," M. K. Wynia, S. R. Latham, A. C. Kao, J. W. Berg, and L. L. Emanuel, "Medical Professionalism in Society," *New England Journal of Medicine,* 1999; 341, 1612-1615.

3. For example, D. Irvine, "The Performance of Doctors. I: Professionalism and Self-Regulation in a Changing World," *BMJ,* 1997; 314, 1540-1542, and "The Performance of Doctors. II: Maintaining Good Practice, Protecting Patients from Poor Performance," *BMJ,* 1997; 314, 1613-1615; also General Medical Council, *Annual Review,* London: GMC, 1998, p. 6.

4. General Medical Council, with its maxim, Protecting Patients, Guiding Doctors, *Good Medical Practice,* London: GMC, 1998, p. 1.

5. For example, S. R. Creuss and R. L. Creuss, "Professionalism Must Be Taught," *BMJ,* 1997; 315, 1674-1677; also their discussion, "Professionalism: A Contract Between Medicine and Society," *Canadian Medical Association Journal,* 2000; 162, 668-669. M. Love, "How Can Med School Deans Reinforce Professionalism?" *The Medical Post,* 1999; 35 (May 25), 12.

6. A. S. Relman, "Education to Defend Professional Values in the New Corporate Age," *Academic Medicine,* 1998; 73, 1229-1233; see also, W. M. Sullivan, "What Is Left of Professionalism After Managed Care," *Hastings Center Report,* 1999; (March-April), 7-13; also M. K. Wynia et al., "Medical Professionalism in Society." W. M. Sullivan, "Medicine Under Threat: Professionalism and Professional Identity," *Canadian Medical Association Journal,* 2000; 162, 673-675.

7. V. A. Sharpe, "Behind Closed Doors: Accountability and Responsibility in Patient Care," *Journal of Medicine and Philosophy,* 2000; 25, 28-47.

8. We should note that the term covenant tends to be used in various ways, sometimes said to be an explicit contractual agreement. For discussion using it this way: J. A. Benson, "The Burdens of Professionalism: Patients' Rights and Social Justice," *The Pharos,* 2000; 63 (Winter), 4-9.

9. S. L. Cant and U. Sharma, "Professionalization of Complementary Medicine in the United Kingdom," *Complementary Therapies in Medicine,* 1996; 4, 157-162.

10. For example, W. M. Sullivan, "What Is Left of Professionalism After Managed Care," *Hastings Center Report,* 1999; 29(March/April), 7-13.

11. Published *The Telegram* [St. John's], February 18, 1999.

12. M. LaCombe, "On Professionalism," *American Journal of Medicine,* 1993; 94, 329.

13. For example, Burnham, "How the Idea of Profession Changed," p. 163.

14. R. D. Gidney and W. P. J. Millar, *Professional Gentlemen: The Professions in Nineteenth-Century Ontario,* Toronto: University of Toronto Press, 1994, p. xi.

15. For discussion on changes in how the medical profession sees itself, C. Lawrence, "Medical Minds, Surgical Bodies, Corporeality and the Doctors," in C. Lawrence and S. Shapin, eds., *Science Incarnate, Historical Embodiments of Natural Knowledge,* Chicago: University of Chicago Press, 1998, pp. 156-201.

16. For golden age, J. C. Burnham, "American Medicine's Golden Age: What Happened to It?" *Science,* 1982; 215, 1474-1479. Although the feeling of erosion of dominance and power is widespread, some question whether it is as clear-cut as it seems. For instance, M. Saks, "Professionalism and Health Care," in D. Field and S. Taylor, eds., *Sociological Perspectives on Health, Illness and Health Care,* Oxford: Blackwell Science, 1998, pp. 174-191.

17. Developed from A. D. Abbott, *The System of Professions: An Essay on the Division of Expert Labor,* Chicago: University of Chicago Press, 1988.

18. The shades of paternalism have been defined in various ways. For instance, R. M. Veatch, *The Basics of Bioethics,* Upper Saddle River, NJ: Prentice-Hall, 2000, p. 52, states that paternalism is the "view that it is ethical to take action to benefit another person for the welfare of that person but against his or her will. 'Strong paternalism' involves taking such action even though the individual benefited is mentally competent; 'weak paternalism' involves actions taken for the benefit of an individual who is either known to be incompetent or who is suspected of being so."

19. New Haven: Yale University Press, 1992.

20. A noteworthy instance of titles providing a particular sense of "belonging" involves the British surgeon, who, after obtaining the qualifications that acknowledges full competence as a surgeon (Fellow of the Royal College of Surgeons [FRCS]) becomes known as "Mr." rather than "Dr."

21. See M. Polanyi, *The Tacit Dimension,* London: Routledge and Paul, 1967.

22. Examples often raised are those relating to mental difficulties and somatic effects, compare, W. Watson, "Psychiatry As Craft," *History of Psychiatry,* 1998; ix, 355-381.

23. Compare, R. S. Downie and J. Macnaughton, *Clinical Judgement: Evidence in Practice,* Oxford: Oxford University Press, 2000.

24. For context and a sense of institutional mind-sets, G. N. Clark, *A History of the Royal College of Physicians of London,* Oxford: Clarendon Press, 1964-66, 2 volumes.

25. C. Rosenberg, *The Care of Strangers: The Rise of America's Hospital System,* New York: Basic Books, 1987, p. 3.

26. For one discussion on the nineteenth-century science/homeopathy scene: M. W. Weatherall, "Making Medicine Scientific: Empirism, Rationality and Quackery in Mid-Victorian Britain," *Social History of Medicine,* 1996; 9, 175-194.

27. "When Complementary Medicine Moves to Hospital, Ethical Issues Tag Along," *Canadian Medical Association Journal,* 1997; 157, 1590.

28. A. Williams, "Therapeutic Landscapes in Holistic Medicine," *Social Science and Medicine,* 1998; 46, 1193-1203; W. M. Gesler, "Therapeutic Landscapes: Medical Issues in Light of the New Cultural Geography," *Social Science & Medicine,* 1992; 34, 735-746.

29. The white coat, in particular, has been symbolized as representing purity and goodness, as well as sustaining hierarchies, economic privileges and status. For recent discussion, see D. Wear, "On White Coats and Professional Development: The Formal and Hidden Curricula," *Annals of Internal Medicine,* 1998; 129, 734-737.

30. It is of interest that in 1842 Daniel Drake exhorted medical students to develop good practice and roundly chastised slipshod offices: "Who can read and think, with method or sound logic, while everything around him is dirty and disordered?" "Introductory lecture on the means of promoting the moral and intellectual improvement of the students and physicians of the Mississippi Valley" (1844), reprinted in D. Shapiro and Z. L. Miller, *Physician to the West: Selected Writings of Daniel Drake on Science and Society* (Lexington: University of Kentucky, 1970), pp. 295-314, especially p. 305.

31. A. Broyard, *Intoxicated by My Illness and Other Writings on Life and Death,* New York: Clarkson Potter, 1992, p. 35.

32. Some interesting recommendations for dress, appearance and manners, in the context of professionalism, see N. Holt, "The Business of Medicine: The Professionalization/Commercialization Boundary in Nineteenth-Century Medical Practice," *The Pharos,* 1998; 61 (Winter), 32-37.

33. Artists such as Pam Hall, of Canada, explore the role of clothes in an exhibit, "Making Introductions." With photographs and biographical information, she introduces health care workers in a variety of clothing, from white coats, to greens, to street clothes.

34. Among a kaleidoscope of images of offices and practitioners, many patients retain positive feelings, perhaps tinged with romanticism, toward the "old country docs," who served with apparently fewer comforts compared with "city docs" with their plush offices and expensive buggies or automobiles. In fact, society's romance with the country doctor is always worth contemplating by practitioners including complementary/alternative. A June 1998 *Life* article by G. F. Dowling "What Makes a Good Doctor? Practicing Medicine the Old Fashioned Way," writes about a contemporary Maine physician "inspired by the archetype of the good doctor who makes house calls with a little black bag and a great big heart. The good doctor is smart, compassionate, dedicated, thoughtful, funny and kind. He cares about all the right things—about love and honor and ethics and community" (21(17), 48-52).

35. *National Post,* June 18, 1999; p. A14.

36. These points on women and medicine rely heavily on "women" in W. T. Reich, ed., *Encyclopedia of Bioethics,* New York: Simon and Schuster Macmillan, 1995, Volume 5, pp. 2554-2591.

37. For example, S. Gaylord, "Alternative Therapies and Empowerment of Older Women," *Journal of Women and Aging,* 1999, 11 (2-3), 29-47.

38. Compare, B. Hurwitz and R. Richardson, "Swearing to Care: The Resurgence in Medical Oaths," *BMJ,* 1997; 315, 1671-1673.

39. D. Berwick, H. Hiatt, P. Janeway, and R. Smith, "An Ethical Code for Everybody in Health Care," *BMJ,* 1997; 315, 1633-1634.

40. C. R. Galvão-Sobrinho, "Medical Ethics, and the Practice of Medicine in the Early Middle Ages: The Legacy of the Hippocratic Oath," *Journal of the History of Medicine Allied Sciences,* 1996; 51, 438-455, notices this in early medieval texts.

41. For one interpretation of patient-centered care and paternalism, Veatch, *The Basics of Bioethics,* p. 5.

42. For context, R. Porter, "Thomas Gisborne: Physicians, Christians, and Gentlemen," in A. Wear, J. Gayer-Kordesch, and R. French, eds., *Doctors and Ethics: The Earlier Historical Setting of Professional Ethics,* Amsterdam: Rodopi, 1993, pp. 252-273; J.V. Pickstone, "Thomas Percival and the Production of Medical Ethics," in R. Baker, D. Porter, and R. Porter, eds., *The Codification of Medical Morality: Historical and Philosophical Studies of the Formalization of Western Medical Morality in the Eighteenth and Nineteenth Centuries,* Volume1. *Medical Ethics and Etiquette in the Eighteenth Century,* Dordrecht: Kluwer Academic, 1993, pp. 161-178; R. Porter, "Medical Ethics: Great Britain," in W. T. Reich, ed., *Encyclopedia of Bioethics,* New York: Simon & Schuster Macmillan, 1995, Volume 3, pp. 1550-1554.

43. For a discussion on the broad meaning given to manners: M. E. Fissell, "Innocent and Honorable Bribes: Medical Manners in Eighteenth-Century Britain," in R. Baker, D. Porter, and R. Porter, eds., *The Codification of Medical Morality: Historical and Philosophical Studies of the Formalization of Western Medical Morality in the Eighteenth and Nineteenth Centuries,* Volume 1, *Medical Ethics and Etiquette in the Eighteenth Century,* Dordrecht: Kluwer Academic, 1993, pp. 19-45. Fissell explores a decline in the emphasis on manners and the problems it raised as a way of establishing medical identity. See also R. Baker, "Deciphering Percival's Code," in R. Baker, D. Porter, and R. Porter, eds., *The Codification of Medical Morality: Historical and Philosophical Studies of the Formalization of Western Medical Morality in the Eighteenth and Nineteenth Centuries,* Volume 1, *Medical Ethics and Etiquette in the Eighteenth Century,* Dordrecht: Kluwer Academic, 1993, pp. 179-211. Baker notes variously the concept of personal honor, an important aspect of medical morality, which we note later.

For the interpretation of "laying medicine open," particularly in terms of interest in ethics, see L. B. McCullough, "Laying Medicine Open: Understanding Major Turning Points in the History of Medical Ethics," *Kennedy Institute of Ethics Journal,* 1999; 9, 7-23.

44. Quoted in R. Baker, "Introduction" in R. Baker, ed., *The Codification of Medical Morality: Historical and Philosophical Studies of the Formalization* of Western Medical Morality in the Eighteenth and Nineteenth Centuries, Volume 2, *Anglo-American Medical Ethics and Medical Jurisprudence in the Nineteenth Century,* Dordrecht: Kluwer Academic Publishers, 1995, pp. 1-22.

45. For general discussion: S. Haber, *The Quest for Authority and Honor in the American Professions,* Chicago: University of Chicago Press, 1991. Also, R. A. Nye, "Medicine and Science As Masculine 'Fields of Honor'," *Osiris,* 1997; 12, 60-79.

46. Differing views between John Gregory and Thomas Percival noted in R. Baker, "The Historical Context of the American Medical Association's 1847 Code

of Ethics," in R. Baker, ed., *The Codification of Medical Morality: Historical and Philosophical Studies of the Formalization of Western Medical Morality in the Eighteenth and Nineteenth Centuries,* Volume 2, *Anglo-American Medical Ethics and Medical Jurisprudence in the Nineteenth Century,* Dordrecht, Kluwer Academic Publishers, 1995, pp. 47-63.

47. As an example, the Chinese Medicine and Acupuncture Association of Canada recognizes the Hippocratic Oath, the Prayer of Maimonides, the Declaration of Geneva, and the Declaration of Helsinki. Information provided to Regulated Health Professions Board, Ontario, February 2000.

48. *Complementary Medicine and the Law,* Oxford: Oxford University Press, 1996, p. 195.

49. Ibid., p. 195.

50. Ibid., p. 198.

51. Ibid., p. 200.

52. Code available from Guild or Web site <http://www.americanherbalists guild.com> (accessed September 2001). Other codes may reflect current concerns with patient autonomy with specific attention to "Respect for persons," "Responsible Caring," "Integrity of Relationships," "Responsibility to the Public," (e.g., Code of Ethics of the Ontario Association of Acupuncture and Traditional Chinese Medicine [2000]). Yet others include Standards of Practice.

53. See M. H. Pappworth, "Human Guinea Pigs—A History," *BMJ,* 1990; 301, 1456-1460.

54. H. K. Beecher, "Ethics and Clinical Research," *New England Journal of Medicine,* 1966; 274, 1354-1360. For discussion and making the "invisible visible," D. J. Rothman, *Strangers at the Bedside: A History of How Law and Bioethics Transformed Medical Decision Making,* New York: Basic Books, 1991.

55. For discussion on this, Rothman, *Strangers at the Bedside,* pp. 149-152.

56. For an interpretation of changes, see A. R. Jonsen, *The Birth of Bioethics,* New York: Oxford University Press, 1998, pp. 377-405.

57. Beginning texts, with suggestions for further reading include Veatch, *The Basics of Bioethics;* P. C. Hébert, *Doing Right: A Practical Guide to Ethics for Physicians and Medical Trainees,* Toronto: Oxford University Press, 1996.

58. *Principles of Biomedical Ethics,* New York: Oxford University Press, 1979 first edition; 1994 fourth edition.

59. Quoted in Jonsen, *The Birth of Bioethics,* pp. 379-380.

60. Manuscript collections (photocopies), History of Medicine, Memorial University of Newfoundland.

61. Compare Lawrence, "Medical Minds, Surgical Bodies."

62. E. D. Pellegrino, "Toward a Virtue-Based Normative Ethics for the Health Professions," *Kennedy Institute of Ethics Journal,* 1995; 5, 253-277.

63. A. Scott, "Homeopathy As a Feminist Form of Medicine," *Sociology of Health and Illness,* 1998; 20, 191-214.

64. The literature on feminist ethics is considerable; the following serve as a helpful introduction: C. Card, ed., *Feminist Ethics,* Lawrence: University Press of Kansas, 1991; "Nursing Ethics," in W. T. Reich, ed., *Encyclopedia of Bioethics,* New York: Simon & Schuster Macmillan, 1995, Volume 4, pp. 1822-1826; C.

Gilligan, *In a Different Voice: Psychological Theory and Women's Development,* Cambridge: Harvard University Press, 1982; K. M. Melia, "The Task of Nursing Ethics," *Journal of Medical Ethics,* 1994; 20:7-11; S. Sherwin, "Feminist and Medical Ethics: Two Different Approaches to Contextual Ethics," in H. Bequaert-Holmes and L. M. Purdy, eds., *Feminist Perspectives in Medical Ethics,* Bloomington: Indiana University Press, 1992, pp. 17-31; S. Sherwin, *No Longer Patient: Feminist Ethics and Health Care,* Philadelphia: Temple University Press, 1992; R. Tong, *Feminine and Feminist Ethics,* Belmont: Wadsworth, 1993; S. M. Wolf, ed., *Feminism and Bioethics: Beyond Reproduction,* New York: Oxford University Press, 1996.

65. For example, Boston Women's Health Book Collection, *The New Our Bodies, Ourselves: A Book by and for Women,* New York: Simon and Schuster, 1992.

66. For example, E. Cameron and J. Bernardos, "Gender and Disadvantage in Health: Men's Health for a Change," *Sociology of Health and Illness,* 1998; 20, 673-693.

67. Carol Gilligan, *In a Different Voice: Psychological Theory and Women's Development,* Cambridge: Harvard University Press, 1982.

68. For background see M. O. Little, "Introduction" [to issue "The Chaos of Care and Care Theory"], *Journal of Medicine and Philosophy,* 1998; 23, 127-130.

69. Jonsen, *The Birth of Bioethics,* p. 82.

70. K. M. Hunter, *"Doctors' Stories," The Narrative Structure of Medical Knowledge,* Princeton: Princeton University Press, 1991, various pages; also, K. M. Hunter, "A Science of Individuals: Medicine and Casuistry," *Journal of Medicine and Philosophy,* 1989; 14, 193-212.

71. Hébert, *Doing Right.*

72. A. Lynch, in J. Crellin and C. Curran, *Course Manual, Philosophy 2807 Distance Education. Health Care in Contemporary Canadian Society: Changing Directions,* St. John's: Memorial University of Newfoundland, 1995, Module 3.

Chapter 7

Public Expectations of Practitioner Roles and Responsibilities

We have mentioned that the way medical professionalism is viewed has changed over time due to shifts in social attitudes and developments in medicine. Many see changes taking place in the second half of the twentieth century as a readjustment of authority and power.[1] This arises from increased attention to what the public wants from physicians and, by extension, from all practitioners. Surveys of the general public suggest its views of the nature of the medical profession differ from how social scientists generally describe it. That is not to say the public does not want practitioners to possess special education, or belong to a self-regulating body, etc. However, it also wants practitioners to be patient oriented. This includes not only possessing the traditional virtues of the "good" physician (e.g., honesty, truthfulness, compassion, etc.), but also that physicians fulfill such roles as communicator, scientist, healer, health advocate, team player, and gatekeeper. Some also want to know that a person exists behind the professional image, behind the white coat.[2]

A real dilemma exists in that few, if any, practitioners can fulfill today's public expectations, if they themselves are to remain a "person" looking after their own needs and responsibilities. As a British physician said recently, about demands placed on family doctors, "there is a real danger that patients are looked on as the receptacles of one or more sick organs, and that the effect of disease on other systems, not to mention its impact on their lives, is neglected."[3] Even if there is some public recognition that too much is expected of practitioners—all practitioners—they still have a responsibility to examine closely how they respond to public wants or expectations, to consider the "receptacle trap." Practitioners also need to be involved in public education in order to make clear the difficulties associated with the uncertainties of medical care.[4]

It is arguable whether current professional education—either in conventional or complementary/alternative medicine—focuses sufficiently on public expectations with the possible exception of communication. Our intention in now offering brief notes on roles wanted by the public is to prompt further thoughts about various professional/ethical issues in contemporary health care. We are not saying every individual practitioner should implement all the public requests, but that they consider them. We should say, too, that a particular issue covered below under one role only (e.g., informed consent under communicator) may well be relevant to fulfilling other roles.

As a Person

Many readers may be surprised that a role as a "person" should have to be specifically noted as a desirous characteristic of a practitioner. Some say it is self-evident. However, as Anatole Broyard said in his widely respected *Intoxicated by My Illness* (1992), "I think that the doctor can keep his technical posture and still move into the human arena. . . . I see no reason why he has to stop being a doctor and become an amateur human being."[5] At the heart of this sentiment, one felt by many patients, is a need for humaneness that may be threatened whenever, for example, a practitioner is overwhelmed by the stress of practice. Medicine, as often said, is a "mistress."

Know Thyself

A key issue in being a person as well as a professional is the ability to "know thyself." To have the ability to reflect on what it means to be a person, on one's mortality and attitudes to others, on biases, on the two-sidedness of human nature, and so on. It is of special interest to ruminate on these issues—long part of our intellectual history—using Rembrandt's masterpiece, *Anatomy of Dr. Nicolaes Tulp* (1632). As one of the best-known pictures within the history of medicine and art, it helps to underscore the role of self-knowledge in health care practitioners as one considers Dr. Tulp demonstrating before seven onlookers—surgeons of Amsterdam—how two muscles combine their strength to flex the fingers.[6]

It is significant that Rembrandt chose the hand for the demonstration, for symbolically it represents reason and the creation of human civilization that raised men above the animal kingdom. Rembrandt, it seems, was endeavoring to illuminate the presence of God in man. In the context of Rembrandt's contemporary culture, the anatomy picture can be viewed as more than a masterpiece of portraiture, for it focuses on the ancient proverb, "Know thyself." Behind this are two contrasting viewpoints about human beings: (1) their divinity and immortality and (2) their mortality and ephemeral nature. While other surgeons of Tulp's time pointed out the mortality of humans, Tulp, through Rembrandt, tried to show the more elusive metaphysical element: one does not die. The sitters are long dead, but thanks to Rembrandt's art the picture continues to exemplify a message that practitioners need to reflect on their own being and mortality.

Much of the current interest in a practitioner as a person arose with public concerns over stress, burnout and substance abuse among physicians. The same issues can, of course, overwhelm any practitioner, all the more so among those who face stresses in their working environment additional to the everyday demands of helping patients. This is not the place to explore how to avoid burnout from stress, but monitoring oneself through self-reflection may help one to recognize when help is needed. Professional support from colleagues must be considered.[7] Although professions such as medicine and pharmacy have set up professional support services, the same cannot yet be said for most areas of complementary/alternative medicine, even though this could be as much in the best interests of patients as practitioners.

It needs to be said that self-reflection does not come easily to everyone. We cannot consider here various suggestions on how to foster this, but they rest on asking questions about oneself and the situation one is in. For instance,

- What is my role within this situation? What is the patient's role?
- How does my role interface with the patient's role? With other people's roles in this setting?
- What personal qualities do I bring to this interaction?
- What are my personal biases and assumptions? How might these assumptions be helpful? A hindrance?
- How might my past experiences be helpful in this new situation?
- How can I balance my professional role with the ultimate experience of being human?[8]

AS A COMMUNICATOR

"Medical communication" has attracted a great deal of attention in recent years, largely in response to patients' frustrations over the failures of physicians to communicate effectively. Communication difficulties are, however, by no means new; since the nineteenth century they have contributed, directly and indirectly, to a growing gulf between self-care (including alternative care) and mainstream medicine. Patients and some physicians alike recognized problems with scientific language and communication. One patient, toward the end of the 1800s, who complained of her physician's demeanor and incomprehensible language, obviously needed care from a physician like William Osler, who understood fully the art of communication.[9]

Communication difficulties in the late 1800s and ever since owe much to medical technology that has shaped changing hopes and fears of medicine. Stethoscopes, self-registering thermometers, sphygmomanometers for measuring blood pressure, X rays, and other diagnostic tools were all introduced during the 1800s. These supported the growth of a new clinico-pathological approach to diagnosis mentioned earlier. Such an approach replaced humoral and other theories about the causes of disease, and contributed to the growing reliance on science as a key aspect of medical professionalism. Almost inevitably the latter fostered paternalism ("doctor knows best") to avoid complex explanations. However, in the context of autonomy and shared decision making, there is a responsibility nowadays to ensure that patients are not bemused by the special language and concepts of both conventional and of complementary/alternative medicine (e.g., over concepts such as vitalism). Constant vigilance is needed; after all, malpractice suits have been shown to be regularly associated with failures in communication.[10]

Aside from matters of language, countless nonverbal factors are central to communication. Facial expressions and body movements often signal attitudes, both negative and positive, toward patients as much as words. Nonverbal behaviors can also reinforce careless remarks (an oft-quoted surgeons' quip, "the operation was successful, but the patient died" may signal poor relationships with relatives.) There is surely, too, a lesson in a British doctor's remark, when talking about his irritations with patients: "they always will *talk* to you while you're writing [things] down, and just occasionally one has to say 'Now look, I'm making careful notes about this complaint. If you go on talking I shall write complete nonsense."[11] This hardly suggests the practitioner pays much attention to his or her communication skills, particularly listening.

Complementary/alternative medicine has also been chastised for poor communication, including the common use of platitudinous phrases. For example, "We really care about you," "We treat the whole patient," "Our treatments have no side effects," "We attack the cause of disease," "We treat medicine's failures," "Time-tested," and many others.[12] Whether or not the assertion is overstated, care needs to be taken in ensuring that such sentiments really mean what they say and there is no sense of double talk.

Listening

> *Nature has given men one tongue, but two ears*
> *That we may hear others twice as much as we speak.*

Epictetus

Although most discussions on medical communication recognize the importance of listening, a tendency exists in current communication teaching to emphasize interviewing skills, or on how to ask the "right questions." For instance, a training manual for pharmacists on selling herbal medicines heads a section on "patient counseling tips" with "Ask, Assess, and Recommend."[13] Even guides to improving communication between physicians and patients on complementary care emphasize questions and what to do.[14] Thus, under "advising" patients, one can read that practitioners must ask a patient to identify the principal symptoms, maintain a symptom diary, and so on.[15] One almost gets a sense of ensuring that the practitioner maintains authority rather than working collaboratively.

While listening is considered a cardinal characteristic of complementary/alternative practice—where more time is generally spent with patients than in conventional medicine—medical education (conventional and complementary/alternative) rarely gives it detailed analysis. For instance, it may not be emphasized that listening should cover more than what has been called "professional listening," that is, listening for information that fits the format of taking a history. In doing this, complementary/alternative practitioners (as do mainstream physicians) can readily overlook "nonessentials," which may be basic to a patient's worries. The failures of professional listening is one reason why patients' narratives or stories attract increasing interest among practitioners (see case history/reading 3).

Confidentiality

Both practitioners and patients recognize that confidentiality and truth-telling is critical for effective communication and relationships. All health care practitioners must constantly keep in mind that confidentiality—long central to medical practice—is a responsibility society gives them as practitioners. This may not always be easy as when, for example, a mother makes an appointment for her sixteen-year-old daughter and wishes to know the result. Are there occasions when confidentiality can be broken? Many will say "never," but others recognize that circumstances do exist, backed by court decisions and legislation, to disclose information that has negative (or potentially negative) consequences for a third party. For instance, physicians must generally disclose information that indicates a public health hazard (e.g., transmission of AIDS) or the probability of a crime being committed.[16] Situations in which judgments are less easy include exposing a drinking problem in someone who relies on driving for a livelihood. Many people ask, Do complementary/alternative practitioners, who are not licensed, have the same responsibilities? Are their legal responsibilities the same as any licensed practitioner? The answer is yes. In addition to a moral duty to respect confidentiality, there is a duty to respect the law unless exceptional moral circumstances exist to question and perhaps disregard it.

Trust, Truthfulness, and Hope

We make clear in the section on informed consent that a central characteristic of ideal practitioner-patient relationships is trust. This is built in various ways. For instance, one issue, especially in increasingly multicultural societies, is respect for other people's cultural beliefs, unless, as many will argue, the belief violates basic human rights, such as with female circumcision brought to Western countries by immigrants from Africa.

Given the current importance of respecting a patient's autonomy and the requirements for informed consent, it seems axiomatic that health care practitioners tell the truth to patients. This is in marked contrast to the time until around the 1960s when physicians often did not tell patients about a diagnosis of, for example, terminal cancer; at least they did not volunteer information if they were not asked. Yet there remain gray areas where telling the truth may not seem to be in the best interests of a patient, an issue of special concern to many upholders of consequentialist ethics. For instance, the "fact" situation may be unclear, or disagreement over interpreting it exists, as with many nutraceuticals. Trying to explain such dilemmas may go beyond anything meaningful or comprehensible to a patient and move the issue into the world of half truths. Practitioners, if necessary, should express their ignorance and perhaps underscore the uncertainty of health care, the variability of people, and that treatment is often based on probabilities. Particular anxiety may exist in giving patients information about, say, terminal illness, especially if they do not want to be told the whole truth. The latter may extinguish hope or even precipitate a nocebo effect that clearly is not in their best interests.

The subject of hope is an important one in therapy.[17] If fear exists that a bad prognosis will extinguish hope and thereby harm a patient, consideration may be given to withholding information unless specifically asked for. Although complementary/alternative practitioners may rarely be called upon to give initial bad news (there is much available advice on how to do this), they are often involved in the care of those with serious illnesses. All practitioners, too, face what can be one of the most difficult areas of health care: making a prognosis. Of the practitioner's many responsibilities, one is not to give false hope.[18] For instance, perhaps to make clear that treatment may not be a cure (few are), but that it may improve comfort and quality of life.

Therapeutic Privilege

"Therapeutic privilege" is a term generally used for a legal defense of physicians who withhold information from a patient, so long as they reasonably believe that it is in a patient's best interest. Unfortunately, the notion of therapeutic privilege is not clear-cut, partly because it is somewhat subjective. Further, it is considered less relevant in some jurisdictions than others. For instance, in Britain where informed consent has been interpreted to be the information which most physicians would convey, it may well be easier to uphold the importance of hope compared with, say, the United States, where the principle of patient autonomy has become sacrosanct. On the other hand, British guidelines from the General Medical Council state that withholding information is only justified if it would cause the patient "serious harm," which is more than being upset or refusing treatment.[19]

Informed Consent

The essence of informed consent is effective communication. However, as the law has increasingly established parameters for the practice of health care, it has developed legal requirements for obtaining informed consent.[20] This means practitioners must approach it (some say it should be called informed choice) systematically to ensure that it addresses

1. patients' rights to make decisions,
2. full disclosure of information,
3. how to ensure a patient understands the situation, and
4. voluntariness (i.e., lack of pressure on a patient, who must be competent to agree to a course of treatment).

A central issue is always whether patients have been given adequate information. It is generally agreed that, for most diagnostic procedures, treatments, or prognoses, informed consent must cover length of treatment, time of recovery, possible side effects, any restrictions on daily activities, information on other options (and their benefits and risks), anticipated results, and a discussion on the consequences of declining or delaying treatment. Practitioners also have the responsibility to ensure that patients *understand* the information, are competent to to understand it, and, if circumstances warrant, encourage them to obtain a second opinion.

Informed consent for very routine procedures, as in a physical examination, would generally be assumed to be given on the basis that a patient's visit implies a request for advice and treatment. However, we have already noted that particular sensitivities exist over examining breasts and genitalia, and it is wise to ask for "special" permission before proceeding to that part of a physical examination.

Precisely how much detail should be disclosed to patients varies from jurisdiction to jurisdiction. In the United Kingdom, the standard of disclosure is a professional medical standard, though this may change in consequence of a new Human Rights Act that came into force October 2000. The medical standard requires that the physician needs to disclose only the details which another physician, similarly situated, would disclose. In the United States, the standard of disclosure requires the physician to cover what an ordinary reasonable person would want to know, including side effects, even if they may not be serious. Neither of these standards necessarily takes into account the concerns of a particular individual patient at the center of the consent process. This is what the Canadian approach—referred to as the objective reasonable standard—expects. It requires that a patient be told all that a reasonable person would want to know if he or she were in the particular situation of the patient. It puts the individual patient at the center. (This standard rests on *Reibl v. Hughes* (1980) in which Reibl, who suffered a massive stroke as a result of surgery, sued surgeon Hughes for not informing him of the danger. A particular issue was that Reibl was only a year and a half away from a life-time pension.)

Practitioner responsibility in informed consent entails ensuring that patients not only know about relevant information, but also that they *understand* it. Indeed, obtaining truly informed consent in many situations is a great challenge because of the complexity of issues and the uncertainty of medical practice. All areas of health care, no less with complementary/alternative medicine, face a vast amount of confusing information. At the heart of informed consent is the need for common knowledge between patient and practitioner, which generally means greater attention to patient education.

Written or Verbal Consent

It is now recognized that signing open-ended consent forms when, say, a patient enters a hospital, is insufficient except to cover the most minor of procedures (e.g., taking blood for tests). Specific written consent is needed for all major procedures. Verbal consent is acceptable for less invasive situations (e.g., prostate examination), though some would say that verbal consents should be documented in patients' notes. For office practice, a comprehensive written consent form, with a patient being given plenty of time to digest and understand the information, is generally sufficient, though verbal consent should still be obtained for sensitive areas in a physical examination, and these acknowledged in a patient's notes.

A potentially far-reaching issue attracting growing attention is whether or not regular physicians have a responsibility, as part of informed consent, to offer information on complementary/alternative treatments, at least if "scientific" evidence of efficacy exists. For instance, should chiropractic be offered as a choice to physiotherapy if consent is to be fully informed? Legal opinion is only just grappling with this, but ethical considerations might well override legal views that physicians do not need to inform patients.[21] In fact, the issue over choice for many patients is not always one of superior efficacy, but whether differences in side effects exist. If a patient wishes to know about "alternatives," a physician has a professional responsibility to respond. The reverse, too, must apply to complementary/alternative practitioners.

Complementary/Alternative Practitioners and Informed Consent

A complementary/alternative medicine practitioner might feel that discussion on informed consent is hypothetical, since malpractice suits have involved few such practitioners. Moreover, some unlicensed practitioners fear that obtaining informed consent can serve as evidence of practicing medicine without a license. However, not only are malpractice suits within complementary/alternative medicine expected to rise, but it is also a professional/ethical responsibility to serve the best interests of patients by presenting all information and establishing boundaries of competence. Particular difficulties must be dealt with, such as the uncertain "fact" situations with many nutraceuticals that we mentioned when considering truthfulness. Some organizations such as the American Herbalists Guild formally approach certain of these matters. The Guild points out to its members that most complaints against health professionals are based on miscommunication that can lead to a client feeling that the expected services and results were not met. The Guild advises on informed consent/full disclosure to create a contract between the two parties. Also noted are positive features such as limiting the liability of the practitioner; a clear statement of standards of practice; and empowering a "client" to accept a greater measure of responsibility for their own healing process.

In closing these notes, it is worth emphasizing that, while Canadian informed consent goes beyond current legal obligations for physicians in the United Kingdom and the United States, all practitioners (including complementary/alternatives) should consider whether the Canadian objective reasonable patient standard is the ideal to be followed for effective communication, irrespective of legal requirements.

Practitioner-Patient Relationships

Any consideration of medical communication tries to capture the essence of what has been described as one of "the most difficult undertakings on earth."[22] To this end, a variety of communication "models" have been proposed to describe practitioner-patient relationships, partly from the discipline of communication studies. These various models, implicitly or explicitly, recognize the issue of power and its imbalance in clinical situations, which can undermine effective communication. They also make clear the importance of nonverbal communication, as mentioned earlier, in establishing trustworthiness.

A useful approach to professional self-evaluation is to consider how one's own practice fits with various proposed models of practitioner-patient relationships. That is not to say that any one "model" fits all situations, or even at all times during the course of one illness. It is largely because no one model is universally relevant that all have, at times, been critiqued as over-simplistic. That, however, does not undermine their pedagogic usefulness in helping to analyze practitioner-patient relationships, and, in turn, communication needs. Again we stress that, although we are drawing on physician-patient relationships, the relevance to all practitioners is obvious and direct.

In 1956, Thomas S. Szasz and Marc H. Hollender, in an influential paper, "The Basic Models of the Doctor-Patient Relationship," introduced three models that fostered academic scrutiny of physician-patient relationships.[23] The models—embracing the "modes of interaction ubiquitous in human relationships"—were labeled as follows:

1. *Activity-passivity:* The practitioner is in complete control and must take over and do something for the patient.
2. *Guidance-cooperation:* The patient turns to the physician for guidance and thus places the physician in a position of power.
3. *Mutual participation:* The patient is aided to help himself or herself.

Only the latter model comes close to any sense of current concerns with autonomy and patient-centered care, which contrasts with Szasz and Hollender who drew on psychological concepts. Later models include the following variants.[24]

Paternalist or Priestly Model

Almost every writer on bioethics says that the paternalist or priestly model—characterized by the practitioner using his or her authority to make the ultimate decision—is the traditional relationship between physician and patient, often implying the "bad old days." Although the "doctor knows best" attitude has long been prevalent, it is wrong to assume that it has ever been universal. Physicians and patients have, at times, always negotiated.[25] Although paternalism is now out of favor, does it—in the sense of parental care for those, who like children, need it—still have a place in health care?

The Agency or Engineering Model

If the priestly model stands at one end of the spectrum of control, the agency or engineering model stands at the other. This model characterizes the practitioner as simply a technical expert who is engaged by the patient. According to this model, the patient has complete power to decide what he or she wants the practitioner to do. With this model, the ethical or value concerns of the practitioner may count for little. When a patient's wishes go against the better judgment of the practitioner (e.g., the use of a particular complementary/alternative practice), the latter has the duty to heed those wishes. Some say, as with the paternalistic model, there is little place for communication.

The Collegial Model

This model falls somewhere in the middle between the previous models. The practitioner and the patient come together as equal partners in an enterprise that centers on the health care needs of the patient. Such a model might also be called a cooperation model. The collegial model, however, goes further precisely because it is collegial in outlook. It sees both practitioner and patient as true equals— both have equal decision-making authority. The door is open to effective interpersonal communication so long as technical language is not an issue.

The Contractual Model

This portrays a relationship between the practitioner and the patient as being defined by the terms of the contract into which the two enter when the patient comes to the practitioner in a professional capacity. Depending on the nature of the contract, this may pose problems because the many uncertainties of health care may make fulfilling a contract difficult.

The Friendship Model

The friendship model has much in common with the collegial and the priestly models. It assumes that the practitioner has an obligation that stems from the personal interest that he or she has in the welfare of the patient. In other words, the fact of professional obligation is not grounded solely on legal obligation. It is also grounded in the personal relationship that the practitioner has with the patient that rests on trust, goodwill, and general concern for the best interests of the other.

However, it is precisely because they are friends that a certain amount of overriding of the patient's autonomy may occur. Information may be withheld to prevent worry and so on. However, as is the case among friends, there will always be a readiness to account for what the practitioner has done, and a readiness to defer to the patient should he or she insist.

The Fiduciary Model

Of the models outlined so far, the fiduciary model is of special importance. As its name indicates, it is a model of trust. It acknowledges that the position of practitioner and patient is not one of equals, whether that be with respect to knowledge, psychological control, or legal authority. It recognizes that the extent of duty for the practitioner cannot be measured by the precise wording of a contract; that the direction of the patient's values play an important role, but that at the same time the physician is also a person with values and rights. Effective communication is a central issue. It is of special importance to appreciate that the fiduciary relationship has been legally established as a fundamental characteristic of any physician-patient relationships. In Canada a key judgment emerged from *Norberg v. Wynrib* (1992). The judgment stated, "Perhaps the most fundamental characteristic of the doctor-patient relationship is its fiduciary nature. All the authorities agree that the relationship of physician to patient also falls into that special category of relationships which the law calls fiduciary."[26]

Barriers to Effective Relationships

It is self-evident that poor communication can be a key barrier to effective practitioner-patient involves relationships. This often involves different expectations about the nature of the relationship, which can shape, perhaps unconsciously, the behavior of both parties. Specific points that rest with a practitioner include

1. insensitivity to patients' needs due to failure to recognize worries and questions;
2. frustration when patients do not take advice;
3. giving too much hope to patients; and
4. forgetting the maxim that a practitioner *sometimes* relieves, but must *always* provide care and comfort.

Patients must also recognize their behaviors, such as when they demand "too much" or have the attitude "There's nothing you can do for me." We must also not forget that the lack of friendliness of administrative staff, especially receptionists, in an institution or office can be problematic.

Empathy

Empathy, a further specific issue in relationships, needs special mention. If its absence is not a barrier, it is at least a critical issue in verbal and nonverbal communication. Empathy, differing from sympathy, is the ability of practitioners to enter a patient's private world, to "feel" their pain, worry, etc. Sympathy, on the other hand, is generally viewed as "I want to help you," but without necessarily sensing a patient's feelings or understanding particular worries. In part, empathy is the ability to listen as a person, not solely as a professional.[27]

Some believe that one cannot learn how to be empathetic: "either one has it, or one does not." Some see it as the gift of most "healers" (see the later section, As a Healer). Whether this is true or not, one can always learn much from patients by listening to their experiences, as well as reading their many published accounts (compare, case history/reading 3). Literature and the visual arts can also promote insights in many ways. The eye of the visual artist, the pen of the creative writer, the lens of the photographer can all stir and foster our creative imagination about a person's feelings. The artist is often concerned with the particularities of individuals, with the variability of the human condition. If "informed" or "educated" imagination about people's problems is central to empathy, then we have much to learn from the creativity and imagination of those who contribute to the humanities.[28]

Many a practitioner has asked and continues to ask: Does not empathy lead to too close a relationship with a patient? Is there not some element of detachment (or distance) required, if one is to protect one's own vulnerability as a person from becoming too involved? Certainly, many practitioners find the need for a certain level of detachment from patients if they are to remain "themselves."[29] We cannot explore this here or the negative overtones associated with the word detachment, which can be interpreted as establishing barriers, aside from suggesting that it is an unhelpful term. Perhaps more appropriate is "equanimity," popularized in medicine through the teachings of celebrated physician William Osler (1849-1919). This can be expressed as: Do unto others as one would like done to oneself. Unlike detachment, it implies that boundaries, not barriers, are established, and these boundaries can be readily adjusted according to particular circumstances.

AS A SCIENTIST

We noted in Part I the existence of antimedicine/antiscience attitudes. Indeed, suspicions, if not distinctly negative attitudes, toward scientists and physician-scientists, are deeply embedded in our popular culture. Issues include a dislike about some of its methods (e.g., vivisection), the intense media attention on the negative aspects (the mistakes and their consequences), clashes with religion and moral values, fraudulent research, and a fear that science can get "out of control." Such considerations are nurtured by countless popular culture images of "mad" scientists who are especially to be feared when they violate the norms of society. Thus, some may be surprised to learn that the public, in general, prefer that physicians be scientists. On the other hand, we must remember that medical advances based on science are constantly before us with all the optimism and hope that they bring to society in general, and to patients in particular. Many patients look to medical science as they do to religion, albeit in a different way, for miracles.

Between pro- and antiscience attitudes, a huge territory of uncertainty about scientific medicine exists in the minds of the public—a love-hate relationship for many. We suggest that what a large section of the public wants are practitioners who recognize that their medical practice is not a science, but an endeavor that uses science. "Good science is necessary but insufficient for good practice"—an aphorism for mainstream medicine—that also applies to many complementary/alternative modalities.[30] Although the attitudes of complementary/alternative practice to science are often ambivalent, by 2000 it became clear that an increasing number of complementary/alternative practitioners had become committed to research, applying, where relevant, the scientific method (see related discussion in Chapter 2). They believe that to gain credibility, scientific validation (perhaps using new research methodologies) must be employed wherever possible. We have noted that a prerequisite for this is basic education in science for complementary/alternative practitioners, which, generally speaking, needs improvement.

In the context of discussions on the scientific basis of complementary/alternative medicine, questions are often raised whether the application of science in conventional medicine is as rigorous as often supposed. Very often nowadays, especially when alternative medicine is being discussed, one hears a figure that only about 20 percent of procedures and practices in everyday conventional medical use have been subjected to the gold standard of double-blind, randomized clinical trials. This figure has been widely accepted—indeed it seems to have become medical lore—although it has been questioned.[31] Thus, many challenge medicine by saying it is not so firmly founded on "evidence-based medicine" as supposed.

It must be evident, even aside from our comments, that science is a key aspect of much professional health care identity in Western health care. Thus, it is not altogether surprising that a U.S. survey (1999) reported that 51 percent of informants indicated that scientific studies were more important to them than word-of-mouth recommendations on alternative health services, medicines, and products.[32] Complementary/alternative practitioners must not assume, as sometimes is the case, that the demand for holistic care excludes science.

AS A HEALER

Patients and the general public commonly wish their health practitioners to be "healers." Yet physicians often ignore the implications of this, namely that they are not necessarily viewed as healers. However, the comment that "conventional medicine deals only with the body, and that it ignores the mind and spirit" is prevalent and must be taken seriously. Moreover, media headlines such as "Healers work with doctors," and "Healing will work when medicine fails" seemingly reflect an accepted dichotomy between "healing" and conventional "medicine." Some physicians, too, who make the same distinction, have sharp criticisms of the inadequacies of their colleagues as healers, and blame a dehumanizing atmosphere in medical schools.

Thus L. Dossey has written, "If our medical schools are to produce healers, they must first stop destroying them. This will require reducing or eliminating the many ways the medical school experience has become dehumanizing."[33] Andrew Weil states:

> A great many practitioners of conventional medicine are very pessimistic about the possibility of healing. That pessimism has many roots, but certainly one of them is the fact that there is absolutely no teaching about healing in the medical curriculum today. It is not a focus of research. And I think this is the greatest defect in standard medicine today.[34]

We suggest that teaching healing—no easy matter—should also be included as a specific issue in complementary/alternative educational curricula. We offer a few comments as context.

Although any practitioner may be seen as a "healer," the term is more often limited to laypersons (at least unlicensed by the state) working within a religious tradition or within a traditional (folkloric or aboriginal) medical system. They include those who practice as a result of receiving the "gift" of healing (maybe, for example, because they are the seventh son of a seventh son). Reasons for positive attitudes, past and present, toward lay practitioners are many and varied, but often embrace faith in empiricism and experience more than in book learning.

One difficulty with discussions on healing and healers is that the terms cover various meanings and ambiguities. For many promoters of complementary/alternative medicine, healing may mean aiding the body's natural healing powers, such as pursuing the specific modality of therapeutic touch.[35] Others "define" healing as attending not just to the body, but also to the mind and the spirit. This is often implicit in discussions on "psychosocial care," "holism," "wellness," "wellbeing," and "spiritual health." We suggest that one common feature of these discussions is a search for practitioners, who as healers, have the ability to be listeners, and who:

1. possess *empathy* as well as respect for the needs (including "idiosyncrasies") of patients;
2. respond by helping to make *connections* for patients, for instance, identifying support or helping with the need to "belong," and to meet spiritual needs;

3. respond by helping to provide *meanings* for patients to account for an illness (making sense of the present situation, perhaps in terms of body, mind, and spirit).

We have already discussed empathy (point 1 under As a Communicator), but here we note that empathy can help with identifying appropriate connections for patients (point 2). Such connections may result from personal relationships (with family or support groups) or from transcendental spiritual links, perhaps within the frameworks of formal religion, the occult, life forces or the environment as in aboriginal healing (see case history/reading 6). Helping a patient to find meanings (point 3) also demands a sympathetic understanding of belief systems, moral concerns, and worldview in general. Anatole Broyard, as a patient, offered one particularly interesting sense of meaning: "If the patient can feel that he has *earned* his illness—that his sickness represents the grand decadence that follows a great flowering—he may look upon his body as tourists look upon the great ruins of antiquity." He added, "I'm offering these suggestions playfully, not so much as practical expedients but as experiments in thinking about medicine."[36]

The need for meaning can extend to everyday situations; one example is when a clinic considered that setting a broken bone was all that was necessary for a boy who fell off his bike. A local medicine man, however, spoke to the boy afterward and asked him why he broke his ankle. The boy responded that he did not know why. After talking for some time the medicine man asked the boy how he was getting along with his mother, for the bone was broken on an area of the body that represents female. The boy started to cry and explained that he and his mother weren't getting along well; in fact, they weren't even speaking to each other. He picked up the boy and carried him to his mother, and they sat and talked together about the problem until it was resolved.[37]

Unquestionably, healing often requires "experimenting" to find appropriate connections and meanings for each individual. Standardizing an approach raises questions, as in one study from a general practice in Britain where patients had a healing session involving (1) a discussion between healer and patient about symptoms and general well-being, and (2) the healer "applying her hands close to the patient and slowly moving them over the entire body while visualizing the passage of white light passing through her and into the patient." Each session was accompanied by relaxing music.[38] Clearly all practitioners, whatever their specialty, must consider the role of healing as distinct from curing, and must determine how best to attain it. Although as some commentators argue, physicians need to develop healing roles to renew their professionalism, many consider that referral to a well-chosen healer (often a complementary/alternative practitioner) is preferable to a medical colleague with similar abilities but "scant time to practice them."[39]

Spirituality

A special discussion seems appropriate on spirituality because of growing interest in its place in health care. Spirituality is intimately connected with notions of healing, especially in making connections to God, to the spirits, or perhaps to a transcendental being. We noted earlier that a search for spirituality is part of consumer interest in complementary/alternative medicine, and practitioners must constantly consider that, in our multicultural societies, spiritual matters cover much more than the world's established religions. Spiritual searches, in fact, range over prayer as therapy, faith healing (perhaps a miracle at Lourdes), interfaiths, and New Age spirituality drawn from many sources.[40]

It is noteworthy that many recent discussions have focused on paying more attention to spirituality in medical and nursing education. This covers a diversity of topics from practical suggestions such as how to take a spiritual history,[41] to a consideration of Peoples of North America spirituality and its relationships to health and illness. Native people teach us that paying attention to spirituality embraces moral values of which respect for people, the land, and the environment in general—is part of healing. The healing role of ceremonies, of ritual and symbolism—so readily dismissed by conventional medicine—is also made clear. For instance, their practices of "smudging" (burning braids of sweet grass with strands symbolizing honesty, truth, and sharing), of talking circles, or prayer reveal ways of opening discussions on matters of the mind, spirit, and wellness. (See also case history/reading 6.)

AS A TEAM PLAYER AND GATEKEEPER

Many patients, in "shopping" for health care, visit more than one practitioner, sometimes more than one from complementary/alternative medicine. This often leads them to receive conflicting advice, which can result in patient confusion and frustration. In turn, questions are raised about the need for team care, as we noted earlier in the discussion on integration (see Chapter 3). However, exactly what is meant by team care needs careful attention. Many observers consider it is more than referring a patient to other practitioners (e.g., from physician to physician or to a wider group of professionals such as from social work, nutrition, pastoral care, and complementary/alternative practitioners). In fact, simple referrals might best be called multidisciplinary care; relatively little interaction between individual practitioners exists, beyond perhaps sending a letter of referral for a patient or a summary of care. One might add, how often does a complementary/alternative practitioner send summaries of treatment to a patient's mainstream physician? Do they have a particular responsibility to send them, especially when they are licensed and, hence, cannot be charged with practicing medicine without a license?

Team care, in contrast, really means a group of experts *working together* with a particular patient to resolve a problem or a series of problems. Team care is not without its difficulties. Within mainstream medicine, for instance, patients who find themselves treated by various practitioners, particularly in hospitals, may well wonder who, if anyone, is in overall charge. Many questions arise:

- How does one ensure full communication between team members?
- Is there need for a good understanding of group dynamics and conflict resolution?
- Does a physician always have overall responsibility for the care of a patient?
- If so, does he or she take full responsibility or are individual members accountable for relevant aspects of care?
- Should a patient ever be excluded from health care team discussions?

After all, the concept of team care fits with legislative and social trends that increasingly recognize a patient's autonomy and choices in treatment decisions.[42] Should family members, and even others, be included if that is the wish of a patient? (It is noteworthy that Patch Adams, in *House Calls: How We Can All Heal the World One Visit at a Time,* argues vigorously that visitors can be more proactive in contributing to health care.) Moreover, team care must be patient-centered.[43] Although reports exist of successful team care, particularly in such specialist areas as psychiatry and palliative care, many negative comments can be heard.[44] These, often as medical and nursing "chit-chat" rather than in published form, commonly reflect differences in personalities and resistance to change that reinforces existing hierarchies with physicians at the top.[45]

Difficulties over team care may be compounded when a complementary/alternative practitioner is wanted, perhaps by the patient or relative. By the early 2000s, many are disappointed that complementary/alternative practitioners have rarely become a formal part of team care. When they do, it is generally in private clinics. Many factors make it difficult for hospital patients. One is that many complementary/alternative practitioners are unlicensed and may not carry appropriate insurance. Also, professional turf issues may be at play. For instance, the push to team care serves the goals of various professions (e.g., nursing and pharmacy) as they search for new roles and responsibilities in clinical care. Bringing in yet another practitioner may seem to dilute professional aspirations. Physiotherapists, for instance, commonly express concerns about chiropractors.

Given all such matters, questions about leadership, already raised, became important. Some commentators, who believe that traditional hierarchies in health care (physicians at the top) should be questioned, consider that leadership should be dependent on the particular situation or medical problem. Thus, the "captain" might be a physician, social worker, or massage therapist. If a patient ex-pects a physician to be in charge, captainship can be delegated for particular situations with the physician remaining the overall chief as it were. This prompts the question: What are the roles of leaders aside from contributing their own expertise?[46] Clearly there are many, from synthesizing expert information, developing consensus and dealing with conflict, and implementing care, while also helping patients to understand any different perspectives about their condition.

To promote thinking about how to approach team care in ways that minimize conflict and promote effectiveness, it is worth musing—as do many management studies—about what might be learned from sports teams and the way individuals function within them. We wonder about soccer and relay running that seem to depend on equal participation of all members (even though stars may be present) in order to achieve the formidable passing patterns or smooth baton changes. For many sports enthusiasts this contrasts sharply with American football with its many set plays interspersed with gladiatorial-type contests, many of which are orchestrated by the coach on the sideline. Basketball, too, is conspicuous for the intrusive role of the coach. Clearly there are many different ways of building and organizing teams. Some have contrasted sports teams with jazz groups in which each member plays off the other, albeit guided by commonly under-stood principles. Even so, this "team" only functions with a small number of players; larger groups of musicians need conductors.

Such musings raise questions about whether health care teams, at least when many disciplines are involved, can function without rules (or written guidelines) or the acknowledged acceptance of a leader analogous to the coach or captain. Are principles and values suffi-cient to protect the best interests of patients, especially if a patient wishes to include a practitioner (say from complementary/alternative medicine) with whom the rest of the team is uncomfortable. It is note-worthy that the tenor of recent discussions, from medical philoso-phers and others, suggests that greater accountability in health care will develop through covenants and social contracts. This suggests rules may need to come into play for the effective functioning of health care teams. After all, insurance medicine and health mainte-nance organizations have all imposed rules on the health professions. Moreover, with talk of dismantling traditional hierarchies, there are those who consider that we are moving toward establishing rules that govern the relationships *between* professions. A number of years ago (1983), philosopher William F. May wrote:

> The medical profession reflects [a] general trend toward con-tractualism in its delivery of care and medical education. The bureaucratization and specialization of medicine today means that no one person, not even a family practitioner, ministers to the whole family or even to the whole person.[47]

These words remain food for thought in the twenty-first century. At the present time, too—as the concept of team care is evolving in prac-tice—every practitioner has a responsibility to evaluate its potential and who should be members in order to improve the health care of individuals.

Gatekeeping

Current interest in gatekeeping—the way patients are directed through a health care system—owes much to the activities of Health Maintenance Organizations in the United States during the 1990s; some organizations, in the interests of economy, limited patient access to certain specialists, and even then only through referral from primary care practitioners. In fact, this is no different from the situation that has long existed in National Health Insurance schemes (e.g., in the United Kingdom and Canada) where general practitioners refer patients to specialists. Many have long viewed this favorably and highlight the problems of a patient's self-referral to specialists as often leading to splintered care, possibly to the detriment of the patient's health.[48]

As more and more physicians become willing to refer patients to complementary/alternative practitioners, they may face a dilemma in deciding on the most appropriate practitioner. This can be difficult in jurisdictions without licensing. Moreover, decisions have to be made as to whether a patient with, for example, intractable low back pain should be referred to a physiotherapist, a chiropractor, or an acupuncturist. Presently, no sufficient acceptable research or clinical data exists to provide absolute guidelines for decision making. This difficulty is compounded by the elusive boundaries of many complementary/alternative practices, in which some chiropractors center their practice on traditional manipulation of the spine and others on energy medicine and herbs.

As gatekeepers, complementary/alternative practitioners are in an ambivalent position. Although patients commonly visit them as primary care practitioners, they may be the first stop in a shopping expedition. This brings much responsibility in ascertaining and then responding to the needs of patients. (In fact, we noted that when discussing complementary/alternative medicine codes of ethics in the United Kingdom, strong differences of opinion exist over whether a mainstream practitioner should always make a diagnosis.) Aside from the dilemmas this can raise, referral is not well developed within complementary/alternative care. It is, for instance, probably uncommon for a naturopath, who practices homeopathy, to refer a patient to a specialist homeopath, unless they both work in a health center. In the interests of patients, this situation must change.

AS A HEALTH ADVOCATE

A story goes:

> There I am standing by the shore of a swiftly flowing river and I hear the cry of a drowning man. So I jump into the river, put my arms around him, pull him to shore and apply artificial respiration. Just when he begins to breathe, there is another cry for help. So I jump into the river, reach him, pull him to shore, apply artificial respiration, and then just as he begins to breathe, another cry for help. So back in the river again, reaching, pulling, applying, breathing, and then another yell. Again and again, without end, goes the sequence. You know, I am so busy jumping in, pulling them to shore, applying artificial respiration, that I have no time to see who in the hell is upstream pushing them all in.[49]

Promoting wellness and health maintenance, no easy matter, is a conspicuous part of complementary/alternative medicine. Moreover, it is an area in which complementary/alternative and conventional medicine can readily integrate. Yet, partly because of the existence of two cultures in health care, the preventive care offered by complementary/alternative practitioners is generally not seen as part of public health education programs. In consequence, we ask: Should complementary/alternative practitioners become more publicly involved in health advocacy? Should they feel a professional responsibility to be more proactive in drawing public attention to, say, environmental concerns about health care? Many believe that to do so would enhance the role of complementary/alternative care. To encourage thinking on this, we offer a few thoughts as context.

Whose Responsibility?

Although physicians are constantly urged to ensure that preventive medicine is part of their responsibilities—e.g., "physicians should continue to incorporate all levels of health promotion and disease prevention into their practices"—rhetoric is often more evident than substance.[50] In fact, responsibility for health advocacy is often viewed as the role of experts in public health, health education, and community medicine. Yet such experts may not be so politically active as were so-cial medicine physicians in the first half or so of the twentieth century. Thereafter, as social medicine merged into community medicine, the latter sought greater respect in academic medicine with less time for activism.[51]

Perhaps greater activism is needed today; after all, estimates indicate that two-thirds of deaths before age sixty-five are preventable.[52] Com-plementary/alternative practitioners can well ask what role they should play. Many already encourage wellness both for patients and the gen-eral public by providing venues for, say, yoga and other wellness courses. Indeed, they support the proactivism in health advocacy that comes as much from lay health organizations as from all health care pro-fessionals. Yet a real challenge for complementary/alternative medical practitioners is how to integrate the same public health issues, con-cepts, and programs that emerge from conventional medicine; for in-stance, how to deal with conceptual differences that occur between a naturopath's perspective on nutrition and that of a nutritionist/dieti-cian.[53] Such considerations may well demand educational reform, for, despite commitment to prevention and wellness, few complemen-tary/alternative educational programs explore systematically health psychology and health education that have emerged as specialist disci-plines underpinning health promotion.

One health education issue merits comment here as a specific ethi-cal issue, namely, blaming patients for their ill health, called "the most disturbing aspect of the contemporary health promotion movement."[54] It refers to self-righteous and punitive campaigns against "self-inflicted" disorders, not only overeating and smoking, but any ill-nesses that can be associated with personal indiscretions.[55] A long history exists of blaming patients for alcoholism, poor personal hy-giene, and imprudence even when a person lives amid hardship and poverty, and, perhaps, disability. However, blaming patients has be-come more intense in recent decades as medicine has emphasized more and more the language of "risk" factors and "health determi-nants" such as high cholesterol, high blood pressure, and sedentary lifestyle.[56]

Unquestionably, ethical issues are evident in apportioning indi-vidual responsibility for the maintenance of health. Does blame chal-lenge the individual's rights to autonomy and privacy? How should one balance a patient's freedom of choice over lifestyle with the need to allocate scarce economic resources for health care? Many ask:

Why should smokers who develop cancer, or automobile accident victims who were not wearing seat belts be a financial burden on the state when many other health care priorities exist?

CLOSING COMMENT

In closing this chapter on public expectations, we reiterate that few, if any, practitioners can fulfill all of the public's expectations. Yet it is a professional responsibility to at least consider how far one can meet the expectations, to recognize that one is unlikely to please everyone, and to acknowledge one's limitations.

NOTES

1. For provocative discussion on such matters: L. R. Furst, *Between Doctors and Patients: The Changing Balance of Power,* Charlottesville: University Press of Virginia, 1998.

2. The list of roles, and the discussions later in the section, are developed from a program started in 1988, Educating Future Physicians of Ontario. EFPO, as it was commonly known until its close in 1998, started in the wake of a doctor's strike in Ontario during 1986. That raised questions about whether or not doctors were losing traditional values. Dr. Donald Wilson, the President of Associated Medical Services, felt that the "medical profession was in danger of becoming self-serving" and "abandoning the covenant of service to society." In developing the EFPO programs, which have attracted attention beyond Ontario and Canada into the United States, much public and other consultation was undertaken to identify society's expectations of its physicians.

3. D. Weatherall, *Science and the Quiet Art: The Role of Medical Research in Health Care,* New York: Norton, 1995, p. 327.

4. For interesting comments: "The sick man asks far too much, he is *im*patient in everything, and his doctor may be afraid of making a fool of himself in trying to reply." A. Broyard, *Intoxicated by My Illness and Other Writings on Life and Death,* New York: Clarkson Potter, 1992, p. 54.

5. Ibid., p. 44.

6. The following comments rely heavily on W. Schupbach, *The Paradox of Rembrandt's "Anatomy of Dr. Tulp,"* London: Wellcome Institute for the History of Medicine, 1982 (*Medical History,* supplement 2).

7. Recognized in codes such as the 1996 Canadian Medical Association Code of Ethics under the heading responsibility to oneself; however, as said, it is relevant to all practitioners.

8. A. Sekulic and C. Nekolaischuk, "How Do People Become Reflective Practitioners? A Reflective Questioning Technique," *Being Well, The Bulletin of the Society of Professional Well-Being,* 1998; 10(2), 7.

9. Letter from A.H. Mason to S. Weir Mitchell, dated January 6, 1892, S. Weir Mitchell papers, Trent Collection, Duke University Medical Center. For a good sense of Osler's skills, see M. Bliss, *William Osler: A Life in Medicine,* Toronto: University of Toronto Press, 1999.

10. Discussions on malpractice and poor communication are commonplace as evident from any search of medical literature databases. Although communication issues center on informed consent, communication is a pervasive ethical issue.

11. S. MacGregor, "Airing the Issues: BBC Radio and Medicine over Fifty Years of the NHS," *Journal of the Royal College of Physicians of London,* 1998; 32, 446-451.

12. See S. Barrett, "Medicine: More Hype Than Hope," in J. M. Humber and R. F. Almeder, *Alternative Medicine and Ethics,* Totowa, NJ: Humana Press, 1998, pp. 1-42.

13. Shoppers Drug Mart Manual on Herbal Products for Pharmacists, 1998.

14. J. S. Lazar and B. B. O'Connor, "Talking with Patients About Their Use of Alternative Therapies," *Primary Care Clinics in Office Practice,* 1997; 24, 699-712. Also, "Alternative Medicine. Time for a Second Opinion," *Harvard Health Letter,* 1997; 23(1), 1-3.

15. Compare A. I. Perlman, D. M. Eisenberg, and R. S. Panush, "Talking with Patients About Alternative and Complementary Medicine," *Rheumatic Disease Clinics of North America,* 1999; 25, 815-821.

16. For general discussion that extends beyond title: M. Carey, "The Limits of Doctor-Patient Confidentiality in Canada," *Health Law in Canada,* 1998; 19, 52-63.

17. Compare E. B. Pilkington, "The Many Facets of Hope," in R. R. Parse, ed., *Hope: An International Human Becoming Perspective,* Sudbury, MA: Jones and Bartlett, 1999, pp. 9-44.

18. For some discussion on this: E. Kodish and S. G. Post, "Oncology and Hope," *Journal of Clinical Oncology,* 1995; 13, 1817-1822.

19. General Medical Council, *Seeking Patients' Consent: The Ethical Considerations,* nd [1999], p. 6.

20. For discussion on the United Kingdom: J. K. Meson and R. A. McCall Smith, *Law and Medical Ethics,* London: Butterworths, 1994, pp. 237 et seq. Also useful for cross-cultural comparison: M. Kirby, "Patients' Rights—Why the Australian Courts Have Rejected Bolam," *Journal of Medical Ethics,* 1995; 21, 5-8.

21. M. Fitz-James, "Discussing Alternative Care. Does Failing to Discuss All the Latest Treatment Alternatives—Like Aromatherapy or Reflexology—Expose a Doctor to Negligence Claims?" *The Medical Post,* 1998; 34 (December 1), 51. See also R. Akazaki, "MDs Not Required to Mention Alternative Med Cures," *The Medical Post,* 1995, 31 (January 5), 10, indicates on the basis of recent Canadian judgments that the answer is "no." However, different views indicate an issue exists.

22. N. Cousins, "Physician As Communicator," *JAMA,* 1982; 248, 587-589. Cousins was also speaking about communication in general.

23. *AMA Archives of Internal Medicine,* 1956; 97, 585-592.

24. A variety of models have been put forward, but here we rely on E.-H. W. Kluge, *Biomedical Ethics in a Canadian Context*, Scarborough, Ontario: Prentice-Hall, 1992, pp. 78-83.

25. Compare K. E. Powderly, "Patient Consent and Negotiation in the Brooklyn Gynecological Practice of Alexander J. C. Skene: 1863-1900," *Journal of Medicine and Philosophy*, 2000; 25, 12-27.

26. See I. Kennedy and A. Grubb, *Medical Law*, London: Butterworths, 1994, pp. 200-202.

27. A substantial literature now exists on empathy. Although definitions vary somewhat, emphasis is on its importance for effective relationships and communication. For some lead references from nursing and physician education perspectives: W. J. Reynolds, B. Scott, and W. C. Jessiman, "Empathy Has Not Been Measured in Clients' Terms or Effectively Taught: A Review of the Literature," *Journal of Advanced Nursing*, 1999; 30, 1177-1185; also W. J. Reynolds and B. Scott, "Empathy: A Crucial Component of the Helping Relationship," *Journal of Psychiatric and Mental Health Nursing*, 1999; 6, 363-370; and E.R. Marcus, "Empathy, Humanism, and the Professionalization Process of Medical Education," *Academic Medicine*, 1999; 74, 1211-1215.

28. See H. M. Spiro, M. G. McCrea Curnen, E. Peschel, and D. St. James, eds., *Empathy and the Practice of Medicine: Beyond Pills and the Scalpel*, New Haven, CT: Yale University Press, 1993; also S. M. Peloquin, "Art: An Occupation with Promise for Developing Empathy," *American Journal of Occupational Therapy*, 1996; 50, 655-661.

For a striking example of an artist revealing issues about the need for empathy see R. Pope, *Illness and Healing Images of Cancer*, Hantsport, Nova Scotia: Lancelot Press, 1991. In particularly moving images, he captures the fears and loneliness of a patient. The lasting impressions cannot but help us understand the human condition facing mortality.

29. For relevant comments, Marcus, "Empathy, Humanism, and the Professionalization Process."

30. The quote, which reflects the views of numerous clinicians is from N. P. Kenny, "Does Good Science Make Good Medicine?" *Canadian Medical Association Journal*, 1997; 157, 33-36. For an anthropologist's critique: D. Moerman, "Medical Romanticism and the Sources of Medical Practice," *Complementary Therapies in Medicine*, 1998; 6, 198-202.

31. The figure of 20 percent is often quoted. We have seen it most recently as a quote from Dr. Bruce Pomeranz, see P. Rich, "Alt Meds' Subtle Approach Applauded," *The Medical Post*, 1999; 35 (20), 6. However, challenges to this low figure exist.

32. T. Pergola and S. Gailing, "The Role of Science in the Dietary Supplement Arena," The Hartman Group Newsletter, *Natural Sensibilities*, 1999, 1(7).

33. L. Dossey, "Whatever Happened to Healers?" *Alternative Therapies in Health and Medicine*, 1995; 1(5), 6-13.

34. A. Weil, "The Body's Healing Systems: The Future of Medical Education," *Alternative & Complementary Therapies*, 1995; 1, 305-310.

35. For example, J. Mentgen, "The Clinical Practice of Healing Touch," *Imprint,* 1996; 43(5), 33-36.

36. Broyard, *Intoxicated by My Illness,* p. 48.

37. *What's Good for the Soul Can be Good for the Body, Too,* Ottawa: Catholic Health Association of Canada, 1996, p. 19.

38. M. Dixon, "Does 'Healing' Benefit Patients with Chronic Symptoms? A Quasi-Randomised Trial in General Practice," *Journal of the Royal Society Medicine,* 1998; 91, 183-188.

39. R. Fox, "Healing Powers" [comment on above article], *Journal of the Royal Society of Medicine,* 1998; 91, 177.

40. C. B. Cohen, S. E. Wheeler, D. A. Scott, B. S. Edwards, P. Lush, and the Anglican Working Group in Bioethics, "Prayer As Therapy. A Challenge to Both Religious Belief and Professional Ethics," *Hastings Center Report,* 2000; May-June, 40-47.

41. Of special interest is guidance on taking a spiritual history, T. A. Maugans, "The SPIRITual History," *Archives of Family Medicine,* 1996; 5, 11-16.

42. One commentator on integrated health care observes "Health care law and policy affecting complementary and alternative providers is changing. . . . A new legal authority is arising which seeks to integrate biomedical, holistic and social models of health care in ways that maximize patients' well-being." M.H. Cohen, *Complementary and Alternative Medicine: Legal Boundaries and Regulatory Perspectives,* Baltimore: Johns Hopkins Press, 1998, p. 118.

43. *House Calls: How We Can Heal the World One Visit at a Time,* San Francisco: Reed, 1998. Adams, who inspired a Hollywood movie based on his medical work, constantly challenges the health care system in the United States. While physician burnout, health care costs, and malpractice are some of his concerns, patient-centered care and humanism are at the heart of his mission.

44. Compare F. Randall and R. S. Downie, *Palliative Care Ethics: A Good Companion,* Oxford: Oxford University Press, 1996, especially pp. 40-59. For interesting developments in relationships between nurses and physicians in Britain, see Editorial, "Doctors and Nurses: Doing It Differently," *BMJ,* 2000; 320, 1019-1020, which introduces a series of articles on difficulties and issues in building up team care.

45. Compare C. Cott, "Structure and Meaning in Multidisciplinary Team Work," *Sociology of Health and Illness* 1998; 20, 848-873.

46. It is perhaps of interest to note that, traditionally, leadership has been (and still is) a role for general practitioners. Often, too, in the past there were physician husband and nonphysician (perhaps nurse) wife "teams"; now very much part of the lore and history of general medical practice, these have all but disappeared from contemporary medicine.

47. W. F. May, *The Physician's Covenant: Images of the Healer in Medical Ethics,* Philadelphia: Westminster Press, 1983, p. 43.

48. For one example, J. M. Lenzer, "The Benefits of Gatekeeping," *Journal of Family Practice,* 1998; 46, 257-258.

49. Reprinted from *Social Science and Medicine,* 37(8), A. A. Alonzo, "Health Behavior: Issues, Contradictions and Dilemmas," 1019-1034 (1993), with permission from Elsevier Science.

50. Canadian Medical Association Policy Summary: The Role of Physicians in Prevention and Health Promotion, *Canadian Medical Association Journal,* 1995; 153(2): 208A-B.

51. D. Porter, "The Decline of Social Medicine in Britain in the 1960s," in D. Porter, ed., *Social Medicine and Medical Sociology in the Twentieth Century,* Amsterdam: Rodopi, 1997, pp. 97-119; also D. Porter, "Transformations in Social Medicine," *Supplement to the Lancet 2000,* 1999; 354, siv57.

We should add that the term social medicine is not defunct, but it generally has more academic roles today such as pursuing population studies.

52. D. Butler-Jones, "Enhancing Prevention in the Practice of Health Professionals," *Canadian Journal of Public Health,* 1996; 87(S2): S75-S78.

53. Calls for proactivity among physicians is one response to changing social needs and expectations. For example, M. Rose, "Lead, Follow or Get Out of the Way: What Is the Physician's Role in a Changing Society?" *Canadian Medical Association Journal,* 1996; 155, 209-211. (For divisive comments, *Canadian Medical Association Journal,* pp. 1235-1236.)

54. M. H. Becker, "The Tyranny of Health Promotion," *Public Health Reviews,* 1986; 14: 15-25; S. Woods, D. O. Ritzel, and J. C. Drolet, "Blaming the Victim: Selected College Students' Health and Illness Causation Beliefs," *Journal of Health Education,* 1996; 27(4): 228-234, p. 228.

55. J. H. Kilwein, "No Pain, No Gain: A Puritan Legacy," *Health Education Quarterly,* 1989; 16: 9-12.

56. For some discussion on such changes, see C. E. Rosenberg, "Banishing Risk: or the More Things Change the More They Remain the Same," *Perspectives in Biology and Medicine,* 1995; 39, 28-42.

PART III:
PROFESSIONAL/ETHICAL ISSUES IN EVERYDAY PRACTICE— CASE HISTORIES/READINGS

Introduction

Part III is intended to prompt further consideration of professional/ethical matters, as well as general reflection on the complementary/alternative medicine scene. We choose case histories or readings as a way of involving the reader either alone, or as a contributor to class discussion. In fact, case histories have long been key learning tools in conventional medical education. More recently they have become widely used in teaching medical ethics. This is despite worries that ethicists may write cases in ways that validate their own ethical theories and interpretations. As stated recently, "Teachers and students of ethics need to become more aware of the constructed, artificial nature of case studies as part of their development into people of moral sophistication and awareness."[1] There are calls for students to feel the "real heat of the dilemma, to use . . . imagination to get . . . right to the core of the conflict."[2] Those who raise these matters may encourage the use of detailed illness "narratives" from patients for examining ethical dilemmas in the way that physicians make judgment calls based on experiences built up from case after case (see Casuistry in Chapter 6, under Modern Bioethics). Fiction, too, is recommended when it embeds ethical issues in complex human situations complete with emotions and interpersonal dynamics. As mentioned earlier literary voices—like the eyes of the photographers—offer particular insights into health care and patients' needs. Although practitioners and patients may interpret these resources in different ways, the practitioner must recognize that patients and their autonomy are central to health care.[3] In approaching ethical issues we have already made clear that a broad and systematic analysis is important. To detail our stepwise approach:

1. Gathering a full knowledge of and evaluating the "facts" of the situation. This covers all relevant legal, clinical, scientific, social and cultural data.
2. A consideration of guiding ethical principles and theories, and codes of ethics, such as considered in Part II. We should empha-

size again that ethical responsibilities may well extend beyond any legal "facts."[4]

3. An assessment of patients' beliefs and concepts about their bodies, their health, and their illness, and whether these differ from mainstream views. This may well reveal why different opinions exist about the safety or efficacy of a particular procedure, and even different views over such concepts as holism.

4. A practitioner's evaluation of his or her own predispositions toward ethical analysis (e.g., toward principlism or feminist ethics), and how these and personal attitudes (e.g., religious convictions) and social biases may shape interpretations of particular situations.

5. A consideration of how to negotiate decisions, alternative positions, or particular views. This necessitates appropriate attitudes toward and sensitivity to the needs of a patient and, when relevant, the family. Decisions are not to be imposed. As ethicists point out, ethical decision making should involve consensus building based on a common understanding of principles and values.[5] Effective communication is an essential ingredient. Some say the character of the agent, the art of the humanistic practitioner, is crucial to medical ethics.

Although such a stepwise approach may seem daunting—and, we should add, other analogous strategies exist[6]—relationships built up with patients over time generally means that many relevant matters are already known prior to the emergence of any ethical, or potentially ethical, situation. We cannot overemphasize that fulfilling the professional roles asked for by the public—especially that of communicator—can preempt many a small misunderstanding developing into an ethical problem. Moreover, ethical issues in complementary/alternative medicine are generally not in the "fire-alarm" ethical category (e.g., abortion, euthanasia). In fact, many issues discussed in this part (e.g., the ability to appraise critically the literature) are seen more as matters of expertise; yet implementing them often has ethical ramifications.

It would be repetitive for us to offer detailed comments on each case or exercise given below such as provided in Case History/Reading 1. In the others we pose questions and offer contextual notes on issues that need consideration. Questions (and readers will have their own) and comments are placed after each case/history reading. Broadly the case histories/readings are given in an order that pays particular attention to the following issues:

- Practitioner-patient relationships
- Patients' beliefs
- Relationships between practitioners
- Environmental issues
- Testimonials and advertising
- Making diagnoses; prescribing and dispensing
- Critical appraisals
- Rheumatism
- Cancer

We hasten to add that while each case history/reading highlights particular issues, these may well feature in other cases. For instance, in any ethical analysis today, it is impossible to omit consideration of the autonomy of patients' or their best interests. However, any repetition is to be seen as reinforcement.

NOTES

1. S. Pattison, D. Dickenson, M. Parker, and T. Heller, "Do Case Studies Mislead About the Nature of Reality?" *Journal of Medical Ethics,* 1999; 25, 42-46.

2. R. Higgs, "Do Studies of the Nature of Cases Mislead About the Reality of Cases? A response to Pattison et al.," *Journal of Medical Ethics,* 1999; 25, 47-50.

3. A. H. Jones, "Narrative in Medical Ethics," *BMJ,* 1999; 318, 253-256. Also A. H. Jones, "Literature and Medicine: Narrative Ethics," *Lancet,* 1997; 349, 1243-46.

4. As an example where professional responsibility embraces more than legal responsibility, we may note that pharmacists who sell natural health products may be considered to have more responsibilities over safety and quality than a general store keeper, since the pharmacist's professional role embraces safeguarding the public safety. See G. E. Appelbe, J. Wingfield, and L. M. Taylor, *Practical Exercises in Pharmacy Law and Ethics,* London: Pharmaceutical Press, 1997, various pages, but see pp. 125-130.

5. For recent general discussion on consensus: D. J. Casarett, F. Daskal, and J. Lantos, "Experts in Ethics? The Authority of the Clinical Ethicist," *Hastings Center Report,* 1998; 28 (November/December), 6-11.

6. For instance, A. R. Jonsen, M. Siegler, and W. J. Winslade, *Clinical Ethics: A Practical Approach to Ethical Decisions in Clinical Medicine,* New York: McGraw-Hill, 1992, approach cases under four broad heads: (1) medical indications (2) patient preferences (3) quality of life and (4) contextual features.

Sarah and Her Otitis Media

ISSUES

- Practitioner-patient relations
- Interprofessional relations
- Shopping for care

This "case" is offered in two scenarios. In each the reader is asked to identify the issues and consider what he or she would (or should) do if presented with a similar situation.

Case A

Mrs. Jones brought her youngest daughter, two-year-old Sarah, to see a practitioner of classical homeopathy, Dr. Kohl. She said that, on the previous day, they had visited their regular family physician, Dr. Young, who had diagnosed yet "another ear infection" and prescribed a course of antibiotics. Dr. Young—he called it otitis media—said the last course of antibiotics had worked, and "so we'll try that again." However, on thinking about this after they left the office, Mrs. Jones worried because her daughter seemed to be on antibiotics "all the time"—at least five times in the last year. She had been talking to her neighbor who said that a friend of hers had taken her daughter to a homeopath because he did not use antibiotics. Furthermore, the neighbor felt the daughter had been having less trouble.

After taking a detailed case history and making an examination of the eardrum, Dr. Kohl recommended homeopathic treatment (supplied from her office for additional payment) and advised that antibiotics will probably not be required. She told Mrs. Jones that antibiotics are not needed in over 50 percent of cases of middle ear infection. Moreover, in her experience over ten years, none of the children she had seen needed antibiotics. However, she did say that if the daughter was not better within twenty-four hours, or if she became worse, the antibiotics might be started.

Case B

"From the other side." Mrs. Smith brought her youngest daughter, two-year-old Stephanie, to their family physician, Dr. Browne, for a recurrent ear infection. "Stephanie was very irritable" and seemed to be tugging on her ear "like she did before."

After initial questions from Dr. Browne, Mrs. Smith hesitantly said that they had been visiting a homeopath who had prescribed a homeopathic remedy. She also said that the homeopath had told her that if the earache continues after twenty-four hours, or if the condition worsened, then antibiotics might be started. The daughter was still complaining though not quite so much. On examination Dr. Browne found that Stephanie had no fever, but that the eardrum was inflamed.

What do you think Dr. Browne's approach should be?

QUESTIONS AND COMMENTS

- Before reading on, consider key issues that need consideration in assessing quality care.
- In both cases, what would you do to serve the best interests of the child?

As indicated in the introduction to Part III, we offer considerable detail on this case to illustrate both a systematic approach and the issues that may arise in any examination of an ethical, or potentially ethical, dilemma.

Determining and Considering the "Facts" of the Situation

History Taking

In confirming otitis media (signs of severe illness and middle ear effusion)—a very common condition—Dr. Kohl (Case A) took a comprehensive history. As characteristic of classical homeopathic practice, she covered a broad range of lifestyle and environmental matters that are rarely covered in a conventional medical history. However, one must still ask whether Dr. Kohl considers the possibility that sociocultural factors such as day care, school, and home conditions (including cigarette smoke in the home) may be, as is well documented in conventional medical literature, relevant factors behind Sarah's frequent episodes of otitis media. Omitting such questions would not be in a patient's best interests, for guidance is needed on prevention.

Children and Alternative Medicine

Any consideration of "facts" must include possible legal issues. Particular considerations exist in treating children who, because of age, cannot give informed consent. Parents or guardians have a legal responsibility to provide their children with "medical aid." If complementary medicine is used, parents might face legal problems if a child, deprived of orthodox treatment, suffers harm as a result.[1] It is noteworthy, as stated earlier, that the British Complementary Medicine Association Code of Ethics states that the practitioner must advise the parent or guardian to seek medical aid from a regular doctor. Parents or guardians who refuse to do so must sign a statement that they are ignoring the policy.[2]

Certainly Dr. Kohl (Case A) has a responsibility to ensure that the mother of Sarah fully understands the nature of homeopathy, how it differs from conventional medicine, and its limitations. Moreover, with a new patient (or family) with no experience of homeopathy, we suggest the homeopathic practitioner might well discuss nonantibiotic treatment approaches employed in conventional medicine (see Alternative Conventional Treatment below). In general, all complementary/alternative practitioners must consider whether they should use (as we believe) a special consent form covering the treatment of children.

Nature of the Disease and Antibiotic Resistance

Complementary/alternative practitioners need to understand the conventional views of this common inflammatory disease of the middle ear—whether or not it is acute or chronic, with effusion or not, the causes (bacterial, viral, and, especially, to many complementary/ alternative practitioners, allergic)—if only to respond to patients' questions. Antibiotic resistance has long been a major issue for both general and complementary/alternative practitioners. Indeed, it can be said to have become a social issue. Relevant data is striking. For instance, antibiotic use for otitis media increased between 1980 and 1992 from 12 to 24 million prescriptions in the United States, paralleling increasing incidence of the condition, which is one of the most common causes of morbidity in infants and children.[3] All physicians need to consider their moral responsibility in administering antibiotics—in other than essential situations—in view of growing professional and lay concerns about "superbugs."

As part of the "fact" situation of the present case, bacteria, a major cause of otitis media, have well-developed antibiotic resistance.[4] For instance,

- *Streptococcus pneumoniae* (accounting—according to some authorities—for 20 to 50 percent of all cases of otitis media). Resistance is now a worldwide problem; high rates have been found in the examination of middle *ear* or nasopharyngeal isolates, e.g., 56 percent, 37 percent, and 31 percent for penicillin. Resistance to other antibiotics is also reported.
- *Haemophilus influenzae* (accounting for 10 to 30 percent of cases). Resistance rates are up to around 50 percent for penicillin.
- *Moraxella catarrhalis* (accounting for 5 to 20 percent of cases). Figures of over 90 percent resistance have been reported.

Any practitioner has also to appreciate that, in the context of widespread concerns over resistance, an increasing number of parents, like Mrs. Jones, are worried about antibiotics for their children. Compliance (or concordance) is, therefore, an issue.[5] Problems are reported, too, of inadequate dosage regimens fostering resistance, as does multiple usage.[6]

How Useful Are Antibiotics in Otitis Media?

Considering the countless number of antibiotic prescriptions written for otitis media, it is noteworthy that meta-analysis of clinical trials has not provided convincing evidence that antibiotics are an effective treatment, at least for an initial presentation of the condition.[7] Antibiotics have no effect on the symptoms of deafness or subsequent attacks of middle ear infections. Given all this and antibiotic resistance, side effects of antibiotics have to be considered very seriously. In addition, it has been suggested that children who take antibiotics are at a greater risk for repeated infections.[3] Moreover, 60 percent of children recover during the first day, before antibiotics have an effect. Another study found no benefit with amoxicillin regimens compared with placebo control in preventing new acute otitis media episodes.[8]

Alternative Conventional Treatment (Nonantibiotic)

Many recommendations exist that children with acute otitis media (at least early rather than later episodes) can be treated conservatively with nasal-drops, mucolytics, and analgesics/antipyretics, along with advice, when relevant, on child care (e.g., breast feeding, pacifiers and nipples on bottles). For a long time, it has been said that antibiotics and myringotomy should be reserved for those cases in which otitis media runs an irregular or severe course, including cases with mastoiditis or other complications, and cases in which there is still ear discharge after fourteen days.[9]

Data on Homeopathic Regimens

Clinical trial support for homeopathic care comes from a 1997 prospective nonrandomized observational study (a surveillance study) that compared the progress of acute otitis media in children treated (1) homeopathically, and (2) with conventional treatment using nasal drops, secrolytics, antipyretics and, in some cases, antibiotics. Various homeopathic single remedies were used (e.g., aconitum, apis mellifica, belladonna, capsicum). For 30.2 percent of patients treated homeopathically and 11.5 percent using conventional therapies, symptoms (pain and fever) improved three hours from initial therapy. Although differences are not statistically significant, the study indicated that homeopathy can be an alternative to conventional therapy.[5] The question that is constantly asked of any study is whether it is sound. In this instance the lack of statistical significance is a problem calling for further studies, as do randomized trials that provide ambivalent results.[10]

Other Complementary/Alternative Therapies

A question to be always kept in mind is, Are other therapies likely to be more successful? To give one example, what if a patient asks about herbal treatment? One answer is that, while there are no clinical trials on instilling suspensions of various herbs into the ear to reduce inflammation, the practice (to be done cautiously by a practitioner) can be helpful. Boosting the immune system (e.g., with echinacea) is also a consideration.[11] While a nonherbalist cannot be expected to know treatment details, all practitioners need to be aware about what other modalities offer.[12]

Ethical Principles

The homeopathic practitioner's remark about her experience over ten years reflects an approach to professional/ethical issues based on past experiences. Unfortunately, no evidence supports that she was up-to-date and took into account published data, such as just outlined. (It is, of course, very difficult for anyone to keep up to date on a broad front, but computerized data bases ease the situation.)

It is also unclear whether due consideration was given—by both practitioners (Cases A and B)—to possible ethical issues. Was there a consideration of principlism—with an emphasis on autonomy, beneficence, maleficence, and justice—to prompt such questions as to whether the care given was in the best interests of the child (respecting its autonomy), or more to ease the mother's concerns? Although the mother's concern over antibiotics (Case A) indicates she worries over the best interests of her daughter, she is, perhaps, also demonstrating a lack of trust in her mainstream practitioner and, in some ways, is seeking validation of this by visiting another practitioner. All practitioners must recognize that where the patient is a young child, its best interests and the family's best interests are both independent and dependent.

Situations do arise, if not in the cases here, in which a practitioner's views differ from those of parents or guardians about the best interests of a child. If any misunderstandings arise, the issues of serving the best interests of the patient rather than the family unit (beneficence) and doing no harm (nonmaleficence) will need to be discussed openly.

The conventional practitioner (Case B) may feel he fulfills a responsibility to act in the best interests of a child by stopping the homeopathic treatment—either before or after reading the studies on homeopathic efficacy already discussed—because he does not believe its value is proven. This may even be the case after he evaluates the studies noted in endnotes 5 and 10. However, stopping *any* treatment in midstream needs careful thought about its impact not only physiologically but also psychologically. (We have raised earlier the issue of undermining a patient's beliefs.) Equally important are the problems that have arisen with complementary/alternative practitioners telling patients to stop conventional medicine, even steroids, without tailoring them off.

Assessment of Patients' Belief Systems

The cases under discussion are presented, as are so many ethics cases, as implying "white middle-class values." Seemingly, no multicultural or ethnic issues are relevant in this case, and there is apparently no overt commitment to complementary/alternative medicine on the part of the mother. Since the mother's worldview (Case A) presumably embraces long-term dependence on conventional medicine, the homeopath should doubly ensure she understands the approaches and expectations of homeopathy.

Personal Values and Biases

Both practitioners (Cases A and B) must recognize and possibly deal with the inherent tensions in the long-standing dispute between mainstream and complementary/alternative medicine. At least, the homeopathic practitioner readily acknowledged the role of antibiotics and had no "objection" if the mother returned to the physician. On the other hand, if the physician in Case B wishes to denounce the use of homeopathy, he has a professional responsibility to take into account the issues we have already considered.

Another matter, albeit not necessarily relevant to the case under review, is whether a trial of $n = 1$ (a single-case study) might be instituted. We do not mean as a "research exercise"—the sense that this approach is often used—but as a treatment strategy for patients. Such a trial is not blind, and does not involve a placebo, but the alternating use of two therapies (with a "wash-out" period in between to compare one with the other), monitored by maintaining a health or symptom diary, can be useful for a patient, and as a strategy on the part of the physician to deal with uncertainty. We have mentioned already the thrust in research to use outcome studies.

Negotiating Ethical Decisions

How a practitioner negotiates a decision (e.g., stopping homeo-pathic treatment as one possibility in Case B) reveals much to a patient about the practitioner's attitudes. A statement from a physician, such as "Well, I don't think that was a good idea," is the type of judgmental comment that upsets many patients who have tried complementary/alternative medicine. In Case B, it would, of course, be tantamount to "blaming" the mother for trying a nonconventional treatment. In other situations, there may be half-hearted acceptance—"Well, it won't do you any harm"—perhaps with a patronizing, negative into-nation.

Another matter is how many physicians will acknowledge their ig-norance about complementary/alternative medicine. We have men-tioned earlier the "ethics of ignorance;" this refers to recognizing one's limitations, and making sure this brings no harm to patients. Ig-norance is, of course, the very antithesis of effective communication.

SOME FURTHER COMMENTS

What decisions would you make about each child's care? In both cases, the decision must take into account the patient's history, and an assessment of all relevant data such as recommended guidelines for the treatment of otitis media. The homeopath, we feel, has a responsibility to be acquainted with conventional medical regimens. For instance, children with mild symptoms and no risk factors (such as day care at-tendance, first episode at an early age (under six months), lack of breast feeding) can be observed, as opposed to receiving antibiotic treatment.

Given all the data, the mainstream physician in Case B should cer-tainly consider the lack of severity of the condition, the implications of stopping any treatment in midstream, the negative aspects of anti-biotic treatment, the clinical data to support the use of homeopathy, and the mother's own decision to try it. In the light of the physical ex-amination we can assume there is no good reason to institute antibiot-ics. However, the practitioner might consider that it would be helpful to add nose drops to the management. Aside from a medical reason, this, depending on how it was suggested, would validate the mother's extra visit, without being openly critical of the homeopath's practice. Both practitioners need to recognize the uncertainties in the mind of the mother and to establish relationships that do not make judgments on her "shopping" for appropriate care.

OTHER CONDITIONS

Issues in treating children tend to focus on particular modalities and conditions. For instance, chiropractic care of children has caused particular anguish.[13] With regard to a specific condition, we mention asthma for which interest in complementary/alternative care has paralleled a rising incidence of the disease, fears of increasing fatalities during attacks, often said to be due to inadequate control, and the belief that patients often fail to follow specific conventional medical directions. A 1998 survey reported that 33 percent of 1,471 respondents in the United Kingdom had tried some form of complementary medicine for their children.[14] An Australian study (1998) found approximately 55 percent of children used alternative therapies for asthma, most commonly, massage, relaxation exercises, diet therapy, and vitamins.[15] Both studies revealed particular interest in homeopathy, breathing techniques, (including Buteyko's regimen of breath-reduction exercises for treating asthma), herbalism, and osteopathy. Also tried were acupuncture, aromatherapy, diets, and reflexology. Amid these modalities, fairly widespread acceptance has emerged for at least some complementary/alternative therapies. For example, growing evidence supports that massage therapy is a favored complementary, if not alternative, treatment of asthma.

NOTES

1. For the United Kingdom, J. Stone and J. Matthews, *Complementary Medicine and Law,* Oxford: Oxford University Press, 1996, p. 181.

2. Ibid., p. 199.

3. M. D. Curry, A. W. Andrews, and H. J. Daniel, "A Community-Based Nursing Approach to the Prevention of Otitis Media," *Journal of Community Health Nursing,* 1997; 14, 81-110.

4. H. L. Hoppe and C. E. Johnson, "Otitis Media: Focus on Antimicrobial Resistance and New Treatment Options," *American Journal Health-System Pharmacy,* 1998; 55, 1881-1897. It is noteworthy that this lengthy review suggests only new antibiotic regimens for the problem.

5. K.-H. Friese, S. Kruse, R. Lüdtke, and H. Moeller, "The Homeopathic Treatment of Otitis Media in Children—Comparisons with Conventional Therapy," *International Journal of Clinical Pharmacology and Therapeutics,* 1997; 35, 296-301.

6. D. Guillemot, C. Carbon, F. Vauzelle-Kervroëdan, P. Maison, G. Bouvenot, and E. Eschwège, "Inappropriateness and Variability of Antibiotic Prescription Among French Office-Based Physicians," *Journal of Clinical Epidemiology,* 1998; 51, 61-68.

7. For example, C. Del Mar, P. Glasziou, and M. Hayem, "Are Antibiotics Indicated in Initial Treatment for Children with Acute Otitis Media? A Meta Analysis," *BMJ,* 1997; 314, 1526-1529; C. D. Mar and P. Glasziou, "Acute Otitis Media in Children: Are Antibiotics Always Appropriate?" *Australian Family Physician,* 1998; 27, 83-86. See also J. Froom, L. Culpepper, M. Jacobs, R. A. DeMelker, L. A. Green, L. van Buchem, P. Grob, and T. Heeren, "Antimicrobials for Acute Otitis Media? A Review from the International Primary Care Network," *BMJ,* 1997; 315, 98-102.

8. R. Roark and S. Berman, "Continuous Twice Daily or Once Daily Amoxicillin Prophylaxis Compared with Placebo for Children with Recurrent Acute Otitis Media," *Pediatric Infectious Diseases Journal,* 1997; 16, 376-381.

9. F. L. van Buchem, J. H. M. Dunk, and M. A. van't Hof, "Therapy of Acute Otitis Media: Myringotomy, Antibiotics, or Neither? A Double-Blind Study in Children" *The Lancet,* 1981; II, 883-887.

10. H. Harrison, A. Fixsen, and A. Vickers, "A Randomized Comparison of Homeopathic and Standard Care for the Treatment of Glue Ear in Children," *Complementary Therapies in Medicine,* 1997; 7, 132-135, refers to an earlier randomized study. Another discussion based on a few favorable results: E. D. Barnett, J. L. Levatin, E. H. Chapman, L. A. Floyd, D. Eisenberg, T. J. Kaptchuck, and J. O. Klein, "Challenges of Evaluating Homeopathic Treatment of Acute Otitis Media," *Pediatric Infectious Diseases Journal,* 2000; 19, 273-275.

11. E. Yarnell, "Medicinal Herbs for Otitis Media," *Alternative and Complementary Therapies,* 1997 (October), 350-354.

12. Compare G. Lewith, J. Kenyon, and P. Lewis, *Complementary Medicine: An Integrated Approach,* Oxford: Oxford University Press, 1996.

13. Over chiropractic management of children, strong words have been expressed, especially in Canada, partly as a result of the lengthy "campaign" of D. Murray Katz. For example, M. J. Reux, "Chiropractors Should Use X-rays and Treat Kids," *The Medical Post,* 1999; 35 (Jan. 5), 14; and B. E. Lecker, "Anti-Chiropractic Zealot Has Let His Enthusiasm 'Override His Judgment'," ibid.

14. E. Ernst, "Use of Complementary Therapies in Childhood Asthma," *Pediatric Asthma, Allergy Immunology,* 1998; 12, 29-32. Methodological limitations are noted.

15. L. Andrews, S. Lokuge, and M. Sawyer, "The Use of Alternative Therapies by Children with Asthma: A Brief Report," *Journal Paediatric Child Health,* 1998; 34, 131-134. See also M. Williams, "Complementary Therapies for Asthma," *Community Nurse,* 1997; 3(8), 20-21.

Mr. O'Grady and DHEA

ISSUES

- Practitioner-patient relationships
- Health of seniors
- Men's health, bodybuilding
- Patient empowerment

Mr. Tim O'Grady, a seventy-three-year-old retired school teacher living in rural Ontario, made an office visit to a physician in Toronto to receive a repeat chelation treatment; for various reasons he found this difficult to get from two local doctors. He had been having such treatments over six years, following some bouts of angina. Since starting the chelation therapy he had "no real difficulty," even on long walks.

He enquired about DHEA [dehydroepiandrosterone], as he had read an article that said it was a "youth pill." The article also mentioned that natural DHEA declines to about 10 percent of peak values by the age of eighty. Mr. O'Grady had tried to obtain some in his hometown, but had been told it was unavailable in Canada. The Toronto physician said some seniors had mentioned to him that it really gave them energy. They had obtained it across the U.S. border, though he had been told that on two occasions at least, customs officers had confiscated it.[1] As a result, his patients took empty bottles of vitamins across the border and filled them with DHEA capsules, as then did Mr. O'Grady before returning home.

A month or so later, Mr. O'Grady visited his local family physician, Dr. Thomas, for a flu shot. He was a regular patient; indeed he had known Dr. Thomas for twenty or so years. In conversation, he said he was feeling very well and that he had started taking DHEA; his wife had told him he had "changed"! He added, laughingly, that he was still dealing with the male menopause. He also said he did not have enough DHEA to last until another visit across the border. Could Dr. Thomas help? Should he try, as an alternative, androstenedione, which he could get from the store that sells bodybuilding equipment? Or, could Dr. Thomas prescribe some testosterone to tide him over?

QUESTIONS AND COMMENTS

- Do you anticipate that Mr. O'Grady received the response he wanted from Dr. Thomas? If not, why not?
- What is the relevance of this case history for complementary/ alternative medicine in general?

Of the issues raised by this case history, we notice first that mainstream physicians continue to question the usefulness of chelation therapy, the intravenous administration of ethylenediamine tetracetic acid (EDTA) for atherosclerosis. This is one reason why Mr. O'Grady found it difficult to get chelation therapy in rural Ontario. Although the attitudes of some physicians changed in the late 1990s, countless others remain unconvinced about clinical trial data of chelation for atherosclerosis, a practice that dates back to the 1950s.[2] This heightens professional responsibility to ensure that patients under chelation treatment are aware of the data, the risks of the intravenous treatment, as well as other complementary/alternative approaches to atherosclerosis. Risk-benefit considerations require even more careful evaluation when chelation is used for nonspecific "detoxification" (i.e., other than for atherosclerosis) where benefits are much less certain.

A principal aspect of the case centers on the growth of interest in the health of seniors and in "men's health," as well as current emphasis on individuals taking greater personal responsibility for their health. These issues, along with women's health—with attendant safety and ethical considerations—are a significant part of the complementary/alternative medicine scene.

Mr. O'Grady illustrates the current concern with personal responsibility for health—at least once he had warning signs—by his commitment (in time and expense) to chelation therapy. He recognizes, too, the growing interest in the male menopause (or "andropause"). This, sometimes promoted as a new "disease," is "diagnosed" from nonspecific symptoms, both physical (e.g., gaining weight) and psychological (e.g., irritability, anxiety, fear about losing sexual potency, fears of aging). Mr. O'Grady's interest in DHEA is more as a youth (or anti-aging) pill, even though he is not from a younger generation with interest in anti-aging hormones. He has undoubtedly read much on DHEA and, although he noted some cautions in the promotion of the product on the Internet, he paid no attention to concerns that it might promote prostate cancer.

A practitioner, whether he or she practices conventional or complementary/alternative medicine, has a professional responsibility to respect the health activities of each patient, and to evaluate their best interests. The "fact" situation means assessing information (some of it very debatable) about DHEA. Dr. Thomas, unless he viewed DHEA as a hormonal replacement therapy—analogous to hormone replacement for women—would probably not offer testosterone as an alternative even as an interim measure. Its currently accepted medical role is replacement therapy when levels of testosterone are demonstrably below "normal" in younger men.[3] Given the long-standing relationship with Mr. O'Grady, Dr. Thomas may well be able to discuss this with Mr. O'Grady in such a way that he can appreciate why physicians generally take a conservative position.

In his discussions, Dr. Thomas might also indicate that there is no methodologically sound clinical trial that convincingly shows any benefit for testosterone supplements in elderly patients. He could, too, make clear that long-term effects of DHEA, if any, are unknown, but that prudence is needed when using a hormone that has multiple effects on the body. On the other hand, Dr. Thomas probably senses that Mr. O'Grady will continue with the DHEA as part of his self-care (or even substituting androstenedione—recognized as a metabolite of DHEA—if that is more readily available to him).[4] After all, at age seventy-three, long-term negative effects from a natural product seem very theoretical. Dr. Thomas can ask Mr. O'Grady to keep him up to date on what he is taking so that together, they can monitor possible side effects. (The uneven quality of DHEA on the market is also an issue, for instance, reports exist that "Mexican wild yam" is sometimes substituted.) On Dr. Thomas' part this would also mean monitoring Mr. O'Grady's prostate health, if that is not part of their current routine.

Although the case centers on a physician's relationship with his patient, the issues about safety must be evaluated by all complementary/alternative practitioners, all the more so because DHEA is widely viewed as a safe nutraceutical.[5] The responsibility exists in providing full information for informed consent. The patient may well want to decide whether or not it is prudent to take DHEA, to consider why it is banned in places. In making such decisions they may well consider the use of steroid products in society in general, especially in body building. Despite constant warnings from medical and sports bodies about the dangers of steroids they continue to be used. Complementary/alternative practitioners who, like others, see this as challenging medicine must nevertheless understand that many patients are risk-takers amid continuous warnings about dangers. Bodybuilders, at least, may want advice and help from a physician and other practitioners.[6] "Your doctor shouldn't be sort of warning you, sort of getting on his high horse from a moral standpoint on this, that and the other. You should be able to go to your doctor and say: 'Right, I want to take steroids but I want it done under your supervision.'"[7]

NOTES

1. This case, written in 1999, reflects a "real-life" situation; after 1996 Canada's Health Protection Branch classified the product as an anabolic steroid and hence a controlled subject. Although the case may well be dated through changing regulations, the issues remain the same.

2. For a recent negative summary of evidence, see W. L. Haskell, F. M. Luskin, F. F. Marvasti, et al., "Complementary/Alternative Therapies in General Medicine: Cardiovascular Disease," in J. W. Spencer and J. J. Jacobs, eds., *Complementary/Alternative Medicine: An Evidence-Based Approach,* St. Louis: Mosby, 1999, pp. 90-122.

3. For example, N. Burns-Cox and C. Gingell, "The Andropause: Fact or Fiction?" *Postgraduate Medical Journal,* 1997; 73, 553-556.

4. At the time of the case Dr. Thomas did not know about the recent research report, D.S. King, R. L. Sharp, M. D. Vukovich, G. A. Brown, T. A. Reifenrath, N. L. Uhl, and K. A. Parsons, "Effect of Oral Androstenedione on Serum Testosterone and Adaptations to Resistance Training in Young Men," *JAMA,* 1999; 281, 2020-2028; C. E. Yesalis III, "Medical, Legal, and Societal Implications of Androstenedione Use," *JAMA,* 1999; 281, 2043-2044.

5. The Internet is full of criticisms of Canada's Health Protection Branch for banning DHEA. Much of this is seen as efforts by government to harmonize regulations according to CODEX Commission Standards, a Food Standards Programme. For example of criticisms see Chapter 5, endnote 7.

6. L. Monaghan, "Challenging medicine? Bodybuilding, Drugs and Risk," *Sociology of Health and Illness,* 1999; 21, 707-734.

7. Ibid., p. 717.

Narratives: Listening to Patients

ISSUES

- Communication
- Practitioner-patient relationships
- Patients' beliefs and trust

We have mentioned growing interest in narrative histories partly intended to remind physicians to listen carefully to patients' accounts and stories—at least for other than minor ailments—beyond the conventional way of taking a case history. Many feel that "traditional" case history taking continues to be short-circuited by laboratory and other investigations, hence the importance of narratives to ensure holistic care.[1] A commonly quoted statement is that an average doctor interrupts a patient after just eighteen seconds of narrative, but that, if left to proceed, this is extended to just 28.6 seconds.[2] Even the latter brief time reflects the culture of the case history in which short answers are expected in response to set questions. Oliver Sacks says that case histories do not represent "patienthood," but only "casehood."[3] Increasingly, this has frustrated patients and concerned many physicians, hence the calls for "narrative-based medicine" to complement the "evidence-based medicine," which, as noted, attracts a great deal of discussion nowadays.

Various roles exist for narrative histories, beyond the courtesy of listening to a patient and respecting their autonomy, all of which can contribute to quality care. They can aid making difficult diagnoses, allow patients to share their worries, and help them to find meanings behind their predicaments, an aspect of healing already considered. Nowadays, in the context of what is often characterized as our postmodern world full of inconsistencies, patients commonly recognize that, all too often, conventional medical histories only tell part of their story;

they feel that their beliefs, their emotions, the meanings they have to explain their diseases are generally ignored.

It is often said that a hallmark of complementary/alternative practice is that it provides time for patients to talk; however, as noted under holism, one cannot assume that this characterizes every practice. For example, a practitioner who measures energy fields often finds little need for discussions with patients. Nor is every practitioner as capable as others in interpreting and melding together both physical and psychosocial aspects of a history; after all narratives—be they autobiographical or written by a third person—were, unfortunately, probably not part of their education.

We offer two "exercises" for exploration. What are the authors saying about their illnesses? Do the narratives raise ethical issues?

Case A: Alice Nowlan and Her Homeopathic Physician

Patients' letters are not usually viewed as "narrative," partly because they are rarely part of the medical record. However, a good number of letters have survived from past times. We include one such letter (and excerpts from others) sent in 1896 from Alice Nowlan to a homeopathic physician, Theodore Bacmeister of Toulin, Illinois. Although a historical vignette, the way Alice Nowlan reveals herself and her needs raises issues that are still current.[4]

Lakeview, Wyom., Oct. 12, 1896

Dear Doctor,

I wish to consult you again about a slight difficulty I am having, and I felt sure that you can help me. I will try to tell you what I can now, and will answer any other questions you may ask. Since I first come to Wyom. a year ago last May, I have had such very hard times with my courses. They are very regular, but I suffer so much and so long, while formerly I had never had any special trouble. While I was home from Jan. to July they were just as bad, so I cannot think it is the elevation here. I have been teaching steadily summer and winter, for two years now. My miller work in Nebraska has been hard, but the work here is very light. However I do feel sometimes as if I were wearing out my nervous system. I am surely <u>very nervous</u> the last few months. Otherwise I seem to be in perfect health. But if any relief can be obtained from the severe suffering which each month brings I want to get it, for it seems so unnecessary.

I am not sure that I can locate the worst of the pain very definitely. It seems to be all across the lower part of the abdomen; mostly in the centre, I believe. The next time I will notice more particularly so as to tell you more definitely. The discharge generally begins at about the same time the pains come on, sometimes before, but it is never free until I get something hot, both inside and out. I do not think it is so profuse as it was when I had no trouble, either. Sometimes my back aches timely with the other pains; and often my head—the top and forehead, pain me, too, a dull, heavy pain, even when the flow seems fully established. Sometimes the backache lasts a full week afterward. The severest pain the last time lasted thro' two nights and the intervening day, tho' I had every thing we could think of to try to relieve me, and was obliged to stay in bed. I know I had taken no cold, and since I do have such times, I am very careful of myself all the week preceding.

I have lots of fresh air, and plenty of exercise, I am sure, out here. Now I want to ask your opinion about what I should avoid. We are in the foothills of the mts. and I am fond of climbing them; could that have done harm? I am always careful not to climb until I feel utterly exhausted, but I do 'till I am tired sometimes. Again, some think horse-back riding is good for me; I think it hurts me. Please give me advice about how to take the best possible care of myself, for just now I am where I can do so. I teach right in the house, and outside school hours, 9-4:30, my time is my own. The dear lady I will board with will do anything, too, to help me. But she and another friend here want to try hot-water injections. I will not do so without physician's advice and directions; and I have a horror of them any way, and hope they won't have to be advised.

I have plans laid now so that I shall not need to teach thro' the winter months, and I expect to be at home after December 16 until the spring. Perhaps I ought to tell you also that I have taken great long rides out here, in springless vehicles, over exceeding rough roads. I am careful now to avoid them, when possible, during the sick time, and just preceding, and I can do so from now on, I know. It has not always been possible in the past.

Please write me as soon as possible, and as for the next time, and I'll promise to follow your advice as closely as I possibly can. Our folks at home are all well. I hope your family is also. With kindest regards to them all, and yourself, I remain, Your friend.

Alice Nowlan

Lakeview, Wyom., Oct. 31, 1896

. . . . No, I am not low-spirited at all. The year has been a very happy one and I believe I have looked at the sunny side of things more than ever before, for I was always inclined somewhat to melancholy, I believe. As to the back-ache, I believe it is chiefly at the sacrum during the period. It was so this time at least. It is just a dull heavy ache as near as I can describe it, and extends from the back through the front and inner parts of the thighs to the knees. Sometimes there is <u>great weakness</u> of the knees which appear as the first indication of the approach of the period. The pain in the uterine region Is entirely internal. There is no special pain in the ovarian regions if I can locate them correctly, and no swelling there. There is <u>no</u> tenderness to touch or pressure in either place. No, I know of no cause of my trouble. . . .

Lakeview, Wyom., Nov. 20, 1896

Dear Doctor:

You asked me to report in two weeks, but I have little to report. I have been taking the tablets for nervousness, but I do not see any great improvement in that line. I think there is <u>some</u> improvement, however, and I rest more <u>quietly,</u> but I still lie awake. I seem <u>so</u> sleepy when I retire, but am always a long time in getting to sleep. . . .

Perhaps I can tell you a little more than I did about my nervousness, since I've been noticing more. When there is the least thing to excite me in any way, I tremble all over for a few minutes. If I know a boy in school must be reproved, it has that affect, even though I am not in the least angry. An unexpected visitor or letter will sometimes do the same. And very little things sometimes bring on a <u>crying</u> spell, from which I find it hard to recover; and yet I am not melancholy at all. I am very happy, I know. It seems as if these tears can be nothing but nervousness, showing itself in that way. It has been a long long time since I was at all given to crying, until this summer. . . .

Lakeview, Wyom., Dec. 1, 1896

Dear Doctor:

I have taken the med. as directed, and am sure there is great improvement in regards to <u>nervousness,</u> and I feel encouraged in every way.

Last Thursday we had a terrible "cold wave" and the unplastered loghouse here <u>could</u> not be kept warm. If it had not been for that fact I believe I should have <u>no</u> trouble whatever. The back-ache and headache were both absent altogether, only a very, very slight pain in the back. The other pains came in the morning, but were not very severe, and after I kept quiet awhile, disappeared altogether. In the afternoon I felt quite well and was not so quiet, and towards evening they came again, and through the evening I suffered quite a little again, but nothing like what it used to be; and on the second day I felt almost perfectly well, while for a while last winter and spring the second day seems as hard as the first. . . .

I do feel greatly encouraged indeed, and am sure you are helping me. Various things have occurred during the past week which might have slightly compared with preceding times. The twitching and restlessness about hands and feet seems to be gone entirely and I think I am sleeping better as a result. Some nights I am still wakeful, not so bad or so long as before—that is, I do not lie awake so long.

Ever your friend, Alice N.

Case B: F. Skloot and Chronic Fatigue Syndrome

The following narrative—excerpts from F. Skloot's essays "Home Remedies" and "Healing Powers"[5]—moves ahead one hundred years after Alice Nowlan. It is an example of a growing number of patients who have written about their illnesses in recent years. Obviously such accounts are very different from those that might be told in a practitioner's office; they are edited versions, often intended to tell of the fears, the horrors, the nature of suffering. However, they can serve as excellent resources to test skills of interpretation. Here, in exploring Skloot's experiences with chronic fatigue syndrome and complementary/alternative medicine, it must be remembered that many physicians still question the diagnosis; moreover, there is much overlap in symptoms with chronic fatigue syndrome and neurasthenia. The latter diagnosis was a consideration for Alice Nowlan (Case A).

In his "Home Remedies" essay, Skloot reveals, in an amusing way, the many impromptu treatment recommendations he received for his chronic fatigue syndrome. The following brief selections are no substitute for reading the entire essay.

The first call was about garlic. The man said he knew how to cure me. He said that all I had to do was follow his instructions for one month. Thirty days, Fred, he said. *What have you got to lose?*

Because I had published essays and appeared on television talk-shows devoted to the subject of my illness, in 1990 I was becoming a famous sick person. The poet Byron has said "fame is the thirst of youth," but this was not the way my youthful cravings for fame had looked—till my early twenties I had dreams of playing left field for the Dodgers or starring in a string of funny but poignant films. No, I had known for a long time that, as Byron also said, fame was like "climbing up a hill, whose summit, like all hills, is lost in vapor.". . .

My decision to go public with my illness was a very conscious one, but it was not driven by the desire for fame. When I first got sick, my illness was so poorly understood by the public and media, which thought of it as The Yuppie Flu, and so mishandled by the medical community, which had trouble diagnosing and believing in it, that I felt the need to let them all know what was really involved. I was driven by the desperate desire to communicate.

Now the communication loop was coming back toward me. So as the man on the phone said, what did I have to lose? He told me to peel a garlic clove by clove and swallow each clove whole until I had to stop. Then I should dice the rest into tablets I could gulp down with the help of raw milk. Since a person in my circumstances can never get too much garlic, I should also rub split cloves into the creases of my skin, grind some to a powder I breathe deeply in, take long garlic baths, burn garlic incense and drink dark garlic tea. I should wear long garlic amulets everywhere. Most of all, what he would really recommend is that I let him come to my house and show me the proper way to use garlic cloves dipped in oil as suppositories.

Within weeks, I was overwhelmed with remedies. A woman who had been ill for nine years wrote to recommend that I begin smoking cigarettes. "I decided that perhaps nicotine would kill the virus," she said, "and started smoking again on the order of a pack a day. I began to recover and it seems to me that my symptoms worsen when I smoke less." Though she said *it's worth a try,* this was one remedy I decided to pass over. Another woman sent me cassette tapes she recorded on using creative imagery to help me overcome the trauma that must be the underlying cause of my ailment. Her wheezy, rasping voice moved me because of the enormous effort that recording these tapes must have taken. Another wrote to suggest coffee enemas and full spectrum lights, which, she said, "recharge the looker." She also thought I might benefit from taking a certain immune system modulator which she had gotten from her veterinarian. *Think about it.* A Captain took the time to write from aboard his vessel near Nigeria, recommending a sugar cane rum remedy given to him by a macumba priestess in Brazil. I should take one tablespoon of the concoction after getting up in the morning. Then, he advised, "it might be better to lie down for an hour. It is a mighty powerful drink." He also advised me to brush my teeth when the hour was up. Since alcohol intolerance is strongly associated with Chronic Fatigue Syndrome, I regretfully set this suggestion aside. . . .

According to my notes, by the time the calls and letters tapered off I needed to quit sugar, vinegar, dairy, bread and flour products, corn, caffeine, alcohol and chocolate. Some of these, of course, I also need to consume to increased amounts. Fruit was out because the worst thing for me was too much acid. Anything that eats outdoors is polluted, so I had to quit meat, fish and fowl. I had to move. I had to sleep both less and more. I needed to have all the fillings removed from my mouth and be cleansed. I needed to see a hair analyst. I needed my head examined. *It's better than nothing.*

There is no doubt in my mind that most of these people contacted me with the best of intentions. Even the independent distributors trying to sell me herbal nutrition products or their unique liquid compound—a secret blending of flowers, foliage, roots and berries of rare botanicals— were probably motivated by a desire to help. There were often blessings; there was deeply felt empathy and an outpouring of personal stories that clutched the heart. Sick people seemed driven to reach out to a fellow sufferer. I came to understand that there is a vast subpopulation of Americans who feel betrayed by the medical community and who seek one another as though they were members of a scattered tribe. Taking matters into their own hands, they are fervent in their outreach, proselytizing like evangelists while expressing their anger at failed bodies and failed expectations of the all-mighty Doctor. . . .

I tentatively ventured out of the mainstream. Over the years, I continued trying everything my traditional medical doctors could think to try. There were letters from physicians recommending additional therapies my own physicians had not used and I explored those too. One considered Chronic Fatigue Syndrome a neurotransmitter and chemical imbalance problem complicated by what he called "an overlay of justifiable depression," so he suggested a specific drug I had not used before. Another wrote to say that one of his patients was helped by a duet of antidepressants taken in tiny doses, one at 9 a.m. and the other at 9 p.m. On the other hand, a nurse who had worked in hospitals and physicians' offices for sixteen years wrote to advise me of the limitation of medicine. She said that I should stop worrying about doctors, purge myself of all toxicities and attend a "Sick and Tired Seminar." After all these resources had been exhausted . . . I turned to the alternative medical world, the naturopaths and homeopaths, the nontraditional practitioners that so many of my unsolicited advisors urged me to consider. . . .

Three years later, I am firmly entrenched in both camps. I seem to have gradually absorbed many of the suggestions my correspondents offered. While seeing my traditional physician once every three months or so, undergoing regular laboratory exams and keeping up with the latest research in drug therapies, I am also considering the most exotic alternative treatment yet: Panchakarma, which is part of India's Ayurvedic, or traditional natural healing system. "Panchakarma," explains Deepak Chopra in his bestselling book *Perfect Health,* is "a systematic treatment for dislodging and flushing toxins from every cell, using the same organs of elimination that the body naturally employs—sweat glands, blood vessels, urinary tract, and intestines."

So it has come to this: Home remedies serve as a kind of mortar between the bricks of Eastern and Western medical practice that provide me shelter during illness. They afford a scaffolding of hope built in large part of material provided by people I have never met, and the growing wisdom to selectively adopt the posture recommended by the Brethren of the Sick around the country *(it's worth a try)*.

I am about to embark on a trip to Vancouver, British Columbia, so that I can subject myself to Panchakarma's several steps.

[In "Healing Powers," Skloot, in describing his Panchakarma experience which was hardly enjoyable, wrote:]

I was a classic case of a person whose mind and body are working at cross purposes in the healing process. Here were these people trying to unleash my body's own healing powers and I was hindering them by using symptom warfare. Did I not trust them or the process enough? Did I want to stay sick? Well, no. That's why I'm spending all this cash. But I felt as though the treatment was worse than the illness, and would end up worsening it. Nevertheless, I vowed to practice discipline the next day, to turn my body over to them and take my mind elsewhere. That was the day the enema tube, on being withdrawn, scratched my insides badly enough to make further enemas impossible, which was not a good sign.

By the end of a week, despite the enema escapade, I had undergone most of the prescribed treatments, at nearly the prescribed levels of intensity and for close to the recommended amounts of time. I left Vancouver having experienced a simplified Panchakarma, a sort of Cliff's Notes version, and returned to Oregon with a recommended program of home care and diet, anxious to see what effect the experience would have. We were warned that it might take one to three months before we could fully assess the benefits.

QUESTIONS AND COMMENTS

- What key characteristics of good practitioner-patient relationships are reflected in Alice Nowlan's letters?
- Do you think the needs patients take to their practitioners have changed since the 1890s?
- Are patients, in general, as knowledgeable today about their bodies and symptoms as Alice Nowlan?
- Do you believe Skloot's experiences and attitudes are generalizable to many others?

- How helpful are such writings for practitioners? Are or will narrative histories be part of your practice, and, if so, under what circumstances?

Comments on Alice Nowlan's Letters

Alice Nowlan's letters prompt many questions particularly about the impact of chronic illness, which nowadays, as probably in the past, takes many sufferers to complementary/alternative medicine. Like many people of her time, women especially, Alice Nowlan was worried about her nervous system.[5] The symptoms she describes—irritability, trembling, restlessness, weakness of knees, and pains—might have been diagnosed at the time as neurasthenia. In fact, the comment in the first letter, "I do feel sometimes as if I was wearing out my nervous system," and her later mention of nervousness, suggests this diagnosis was probably on her mind.[6] Neurasthenia was the diagnostic label, which emerged in the last decades of the nineteenth century, to describe a state of "physical" and "mental exhaustion," characterized by often vague symptoms. Although the symptomatology fits menstrual discomfort, menstruation and nervousness were closely associated in defining the biology of women.

In Alice Nowlan's letters no evidence exists that the precise diagnostic label was used; perhaps, this reflected the homeopathic approach to treatment (with an emphasis on patterns of symptoms) or a reluctance—as among some practitioners today—to legitimize a condition with diverse and inconsistent symptoms by labeling it. Certainly Alice Nowlan was left with various possibilities to account for her condition from the climate to horse riding. Her search for an explanation is obvious, as is her faith in her physician. Indeed trust is a key characteristic evident in the letters, a characteristic considered to be at the heart of practitioner-patient relationships as noted earlier. At the same time, it is evident that she was taking responsibility for her health at a time when women were commonly viewed as being controlled by the biology of their bodies.

Comments on F. Skloot and Chronic Fatigue Syndrome

The second narrative—one written for public consumption—has obviously a different purpose. Nevertheless, do similarities exist?

Skloot is an accomplished author with a readership to cultivate and consider. He does this through exploring diverse aspects of his illness. In part this is for him a form of therapy. As he wrote:

> Oliver Sacks says that "to be ourselves we must have ourselves—possess if need be, repossess our life-stories. We must 'recollect' ourselves, recollect the inner drama, the narrative, ourselves." This is what we need to hold on to, by hook or by crook, if we are to keep whole. We usually tell our stories only to our physicians, loved ones, or friends. Perhaps we should begin telling it more widely, in chat rooms, in groups, onto tape, in writing. By telling, we not only help ourselves remember, we educate, we bear witness and we claim our humanity.[7]

Few readers can disagree that Skloot's writings illustrate this, as he offers many insights into feelings and attitudes. For instance, after his account of the diversity of recommended treatments (which is certainly the experience of others), he comments on a dilemma facing many people "trying out" complementary/alternative medicine, but with a little skepticism. Among insights Skloot offers about illness and treatment, he raises, in an interesting way, the role of belief when he talks of his mind and body "working at cross purposes in the healing process."

The importance of belief and trust in health care has received much attention in recent times, especially in connection with the placebo effect (see Efficacy, Effectiveness, and Placebos in Chapter 4). It is often said that belief is particularly relevant in complementary/alternative care, because of a patient's investment of personal responsibility. As some say, perhaps, a patient's failure to believe deeply enough or failure to eliminate negative thinking is at fault when the disease gets worse. "The system did not fail; I did."[8]

We strongly recommend Skloot's writings. The circumstances he describes are by no means unique and they offer practitioners many insights into suffering from chronic conditions.

NOTES

1. M. G. Nagai-Jacobson and M. A. Burkhardt, "Viewing Persons As Stories: A Perspective for Holistic Care," *Alternative Therapies in Health and Medicine,* 1996; 2(4), 54-58.

2. Quoted, for instance, in P. Dieppe, "Narrative Based Medicine," *Journal Royal Society of Medicine,* 1999; 92, 380-381.

3. O. Sacks, "Clinical Tales," *Literature and Medicine,* 1986; 5, 16-23.

4. For background and information on Bacmeister, J. K. Crellin, *Medical Care in Pioneer Illinois,* Springfield: Pearson Museum, SIU Medical School (Medical Humanities Series), 1982, pp. 79-82.

5. The essays appear in *The Night-Side: Chronic Fatigue Syndrome and the Illness Experience,* Brownsville: Story Line Press, 1996, pp. 105-118, 119-131.

6. The issue of nervousness was widespread at the time of the letters. Compare J. Oppenheim, *"Shattered Nerves": Doctors, Patients and Depression in Victorian England,* New York: Oxford University Press, 1991; although dealing with Britain, Oppenheim's story has many parallels with the United States.

7. <http://www.oregonlive.com/books/nov/BK971126BS.html> (accessed September 20, 2001).

8. F. Davidoff, "Weighing the Alternatives: Lessons from the Paradoxes of Alternative Medicine," *Annals of Internal Medicine,* 1998; 129, 1068-1070, quoting T. J. Kaptchuk and D. M. Eisenberg, "The Persuasive Appeal of Alternative Medicine," Annals of Internal Medicine, 1998; 129, 1061-1065.

– 4 –

Difficult Professional Relationships

ISSUES

- Interprofessional relationships
- Whistle-blowing
- Practitioner-patient relationships
- Ethics of ignorance

Case A: Homeopathy—A Pharmacist's Dilemma

Pharmacist Craig Stadler spoke with Mr. Montrose, who has just been admitted to the Catholic hospital in a large midwestern U.S. town for an elective surgical procedure. In taking a drug history, Stadler found that Mr. Montrose takes a homeopathic preparation, recommended by Dr. Allen, a staff physician, for allergies. Mr. Montrose asked, "What is your advice about homeopathy? I think it helps, but I haven't been able to find anything about this homeopathic one in the references I got from the library."

Pharmacist Stadler stated he did not believe in homeopathy and that pharmacists generally feel that it is unscientific and hence unethical. If it "works" at all it is because of placebo effect. He has heard that Dr. Allen truly believes in the efficacy of some homeopathic remedies. Although he has never met Dr. Allen, Stadler thinks that anyone who prescribes such preparations is a charlatan, as he told Mr. Montrose; he also said that Dr. Allen hailed from Europe and was old-fashioned. He concluded, "We now know that homeopathy is unscientific and you should stick to regular medicine."[1]

Case B: A Telephone Conversation

Mrs. Smith telephoned Dr. Ross, a chiropractor who had been treating her sister. She had concerns about another chiropractor, "Dr. King in the shopping mall," after she visited him with her son. She had been told that he could cure her son's asthma, but that if she did not bring him regularly he would "become chronically sick."

Dr. Ross said it was an unfortunate comment that sounded very unprofessional. He told Mrs. Smith that she could make a complaint to the state licensing board if she wished.

Mrs. Smith then asked, "Can you cure him?" Ross explained that in reality no practitioner "cures," and that it is difficult to discuss such matters over the phone without knowing details of her son's problem. He asked if she had any specific questions? In fact, she asked about a herbal medicine she had been taking herself. It had been suggested by a friend and she was not sure what it was. Also, she thought it made her anxious. Ross recommended that she stop taking the herbal remedy and come to see him, with her son, as soon as possible.

On putting down the phone, Ross wondered whether he should have suggested that Mrs. Smith complain to the licensing board. On the other hand, he had heard of a number of negative comments about Dr. King during the past year. Should he discuss this with the board?

QUESTIONS AND COMMENTS

- What professional/ethical issues do you see in the "cases"?
- Would you consider a complaint to a disciplinary board?

Case A

Although the case offers "honest opinions" about another health professional, does it constitute "bad mouthing"? Depending on circumstances, this can have many implications for a patient's peace of mind, and on efforts to integrate his or her own care.

The "facts" of the situation are straightforward, at least for pharmacist Stadler. He follows long-standing negative thinking about homeopathy among pharmacists, albeit being moderated in recent years. For instance:

> We urge pharmacists not to stock homeopathic remedies and to inform customers that such products simply don't work. We also hope that pharmacy educators, journal editors, and pharmacy organizations will regard this as an important ethical issue.[2]

Stadler undoubtedly accepted, without firsthand knowledge of published studies and without clinical evidence, the widely held view that it is incomprehensible that dilute homeopathic preparations could have any physiological effect.

In turning to our systematic approach to any case, we must ask whether pharmacist Stadler needs to ask himself whether he has all the "facts," can be said to be biased, and whether the ethics of ignorance is relevant. As we have discussed, lack of facts can lead to poor judgments and hence create unnecessary ethical issues. Certainly Stadler is unaware of homeopathy's reputation in treating allergies. Does he not have a responsibility to explore with Mr. Montrose the disagreements that exist over homeopathy? After all, he has been asked for advice, not opinion. He might suggest that Mr. Montrose ask Dr. Allen about suitable reading. Stadler must consider carefully the meanings of being scientific and unscientific, recognize personal biases, and place the best interests of the patient at the center of decision making.

With regard to Mr. Montrose's best interests, although we do not know if he had been trying homeopathic care for some time and whether the allergies had been helped by the homeopathy, it does not appear that he is committed to homeopathy. However, Stadler needs to appreciate a professional responsibility not to undermine a patient's confidence in his or her existing regimen unless it is known to be unsafe.

Case B

The Mrs. Smith case, which also dealt with relationships to another health professional, raises questions about whistle-blowing, although, as is often the case, the situation is not clear-cut. The comments about curing asthma and "chronic sickness" may be a misunderstanding; on the other hand, a pattern of concerns seems to be arising.

The issue of whistle-blowing has become more prominent in recent years, in part a reaction to the view that the medical profession has long protected its own. Despite recent high profile cases of dangerous clinical practice by physicians that have put the profession on the defensive, questions arise whether silence still occurs.

Particular difficulties can arise for the whistle-blower. Do elements of revenge or of gain play a part in making accusations? How does one deal with breeching loyalty to a colleague? Will nurses who accuse physicians of bad practice be seen as troublemakers? The problems facing whistle-blowing physicians and nurses are well documented. For nurses, in particular, their professional ethic of being a patient advocate adds to difficulties.

Most problems have arisen over alcoholism, drug abuse, and stress-related behavior. Professional bodies in medicine, nursing, and other mainstream health professions have established treatment centers for their members which will protect confidentiality. Unfortunately, this is currently beyond the capability of complementary/alternative medical organizations, although much anecdotal evidence indicates that problems exist as much among complementary/alternative practitioners as among mainstream practitioners. Further, the absence of licensing in many jurisdictions means that no effective mechanism is available for hearing patients' complaints or disciplining practitioners.

Another issue in Case B involves telephone consultation. It is often said that complementary/alternative practitioners are, generally speaking, more available over the phone than are mainstream practitioners. After all, most complementary practitioners must promote and/or make themselves more available to the public. Failure to do so may have negative consequences on building up a practice. Yet telephone advice obviously has many pitfalls, and particular care must be taken to limit its scope and to ensure that communication has been effective.

NOTES

1. Adapted from a case in "Informing a Patient About a Homeopathic Preparation," *American Journal of Health-System Pharmacy,* 1995; 52, 2437-2441.

2. S. Barrett and V. E. Tyler, "Why Pharmacists Should Not Sell Homeopathic Remedies," *American Journal of Health-System Pharmacy,* 1995; 52, 1004-1006; for further discussion, J. K. Crellin, "Alternative Medicine Ethical Challenges for the Profession of Pharmacy," in J. M. Humber and R. F. Almeder, eds., *Alternative Medicine and Ethics,* Totowa, NJ: Humana Press, 1998, pp. 195-212.

–5–

Mr. L: The Dilemmas
of Multicultural Health

ISSUES

- Patients' beliefs
- Multicultural health issues
- Team care
- Integrated care

In our increasingly multicultural Western societies many health practitioners face difficulties with patients' beliefs that differ from their own. Conventional physicians often see this translated into demands for unfamiliar treatments. Complementary/alternative practitioners may believe they are more sensitive to nonmainstream beliefs, but generally they face the same learning curve about other cultures. What approaches should one take? What attitudes should one take toward cultural relativism?

Considerable discussion has appeared regarding Hmong refugees from North Vietnam, in Western countries (over 100,000 are present in the United States). It is clear that very significant differences in the health beliefs exist between them and Western-trained, mainstream practitioners. At the same time practitioners need to uncover and understand the particular attitudes and beliefs of an *individual* patient, for it is always dangerous to stereotype every person in an ethnic group as holding the same beliefs and customs. A strong case invariably exists for developing a narrative history. We cannot include a lengthy narrative here but have summarized an important account, published in 1995, about the medical history of a Hmong patient.[1] Unlike the narratives in case history/reading 3, it is written by an "observer" (a nonphysician). It must be recognized that such third-person narratives—more often developed by practitioners—have the inherent danger of incorporating the narrator's interpretations and biases.

The Case of Mr. L

The narrator first provided a brief biography and how Mr. L arrived in Philadelphia. Then "In October 1987, Mr. L became ill suddenly and began to vomit blood. Family members took him to the emergency room of a large local teaching hospital. He was shortly diagnosed as being in incipient liver failure as a result of liver tissue damage caused by chronic hepatitis B. He was admitted to the hospital on an emergency basis." His condition was discussed in detail as well as the arrangements for evaluation for a liver transplant, and treatment of the associated esophageal varices with sclerotherapy. The narrator states that in Mr. L's case, all of the interactions were complicated by cultural differences between conventional medical and Hmong views over the nature of sickness and of emergency, of the time requirement needed to make decisions, of the different approaches to selecting appropriate times for action, of dietary requirements, of the different views over proper treatment and of risk, and of what is acceptable in handling the body. Further, Mr. L had never been in a hospital, and his family members were entirely unfamiliar with the complexity of hospital life.

Of special concern for Mr. L and his family was the bleeding episode, but seemingly it was interpreted as an isolated serious incident of unknown cause, rather than the hospital physicians' diagnosis that it was symptomatic of a serious underlying disease of long duration. Further, Mr. L's only complaint at the time of his crisis, other than the bleeding, was fatigue. His ascites, associated with the liver dysfunction, tended to be interpreted by the Hmong community as visible effects of fat "regarded as one of two essential elements (together with blood) that provide vitality to the body."

Mr. L's hospitalization ended with the family's decision to reject the option of a liver transplant, and to refuse further evaluation. "Though some of the younger men in the family felt that the evaluation itself could do no harm, the older men (and in general the majority of the decision-making body) felt that pursuit of the evaluation would involve a significant risk of being coerced by the physicians."

Mr. L left the hospital against medical advice, and went home with some prophylactic care.

The family did get a second opinion from a physician who approached Mr. L more conservatively and outlined a much longer time frame for decision making than the rush established by the previous doctor. Unfortunately, possibly because of missing some sclerotherapy sessions intended to prevent a recurrence of bleeding, Mr. L suffered a second bleeding episode, and was admitted to the medical Intensive Care Unit where considerable effort was required to stabilize him. Ultimately he was transferred to a surgical floor of the hospital, a floor unfamiliar to him where he faced physicians whom he had never met. "These strangers strongly recommended that he undergo surgery for the placement of a venous shunt, a device designed to decrease the likelihood of rebleeding of the esophageal varices." The proposal, which offered an internal mechanism to control Mr. L's bleeding varices, addressed the physicians' concern that this "uncooperative patient" might again fail to adhere to the rather difficult medical regimen thus causing dangerous (and possibly fatal) results.

Again, Mr. L was presented with consent forms and pressured to make a decision. The surgeons considered that the decision in favor of the shunt had already been made; "the scheduling of the surgery and its preliminary procedures (including an angiogram, terrifying to Mr. L in its own right) waited only for the patient to catch up to the decision." Although the Hmong patterns of decision making had become part of Mr. L's medical record, and the medical and nursing staff made genuine efforts to respect them, the staff were frustrated by the different senses of urgency between themselves and Mr. L. The nurses requested a patient-care conference focusing on cultural issues, and were extremely accommodating of Mr. L's special needs. They gave him detailed explanations of all procedures proposed, illustrating their explanations with photographs and diagrams from anatomy books. "They arranged for the hospital kitchen to prepare ricewater for him, as his regimen once again restricted him to clear liquids, and this generous step helped to relieve one genuine source of suffering: being forbidden to eat rice." Mr. L appreciated these efforts, but remained resistant to the pressure that was coercing him to reach a conforming decision about the proposed surgery.

Mr. L would not make a decision without consulting his more conservative doctor, with the result that conservative treatment was continued with a commitment by Mr. L that he would strictly follow the regimen laid out for him. With this, in addition to observing traditional Hmong religious practices and herbal medications as preventive health measures, Mr. L was leading a full and active life at the time of the publication of the narrative.

QUESTIONS AND COMMENTS

- What cultural considerations are relevant to quality care?
- Did Mr. L receive appropriate "team care"?
- Are terms such as "uncooperative patient" appropriate?
- What are some key ethical issues in multicultural health?

Apart from highlighting health care issues that can arise in our increasingly pluralistic societies, the case contrasts two treatment philosophies in mainstream medicine. These—proactive and conservative—remind us of the importance of considering how best to accommodate different beliefs and needs. However, to what extent can all beliefs be accepted by practitioners? Cultural pluralism offers numerous challenges that impinge on health matters. Generally speaking, all cultural practices should be respected. However, few condone—albeit amid much ethical debate—those that violate human rights, such as female circumcision, a cultural practice brought to Western countries by African immigrants. In other words, cultural relativism is generally accepted to have limits when one culture is transplanted into another. Defining these limits is not easy, but at least some justification can be found for seeing the humanity and humaneness of the dominant culture as overriding cultural sensitivities.

Even practitioners who are sensitive to cultural relativism may overlook ways in which cultural sensitivities are overridden. For instance, can the commitment to respecting a patient's autonomy discriminate against those who do not wish to be told bad news? This was an issue in Mr. L's case; it is unclear whether he really wished to be told in detail exactly what his problems were, or whether he was able to comprehend the information.

The term cultural competency has emerged to describe whether a practitioner has sufficient education, knowledge, and skills to understand the particular needs and concerns of patients from different ethnic backgrounds and different countries. It is clear that in Mr. L's first emergency he met a physician who apparently lacked this professional requirement. Unquestionably, cultural competency is necessary to provide quality care, to respect the autonomy of a patient (that is as he or she sees autonomy), to elicit true informed consent, and perhaps to negotiate a regimen that both practitioner and patient see as being in their best interests.

NOTE

1. B. B. O'Connor, *Healing Traditions, Alternative Medicine and the Health Professions,* Philadelphia: University of Pennsylvania Press, 1995, pp. 82-104.

The Environment and Connections

ISSUES

- To what extent does the environment contribute to health care?
- What responsibilities do practitioners have to promote environmental concerns?
- Environmental ethics.

A professional issue for all practitioners is to decide on their responsibilities toward the environment and the extent to which these responsibilities can be fulfilled (see Chapter 7). Naturally, this demands an awareness of public attitudes and beliefs. In offering further comments we begin with (a) some remarks on "Ceremonies link us with the environment" by the chief of a Mi'kmaq band in Canada,[1] and (b) a brief outline of a case.

Case A: Chief Misel Joe Discusses Healing Ceremonies

Sweatlodge ceremonies are one way we find that helps to bring young and old together, to talk about the alcoholism, to talk about family abuse, to talk about verbal abuse which is sometimes very common in aboriginal communities. And in the sweatlodge ceremony, we talk about how that's not acceptable, and how verbal abuse can have long lasting effects on an individual.

The other ceremonies that we do every time we meet is to have a sweetgrass ceremony, a purification ceremony. The purpose for the sweetgrass ceremony is to ask each other to have respect for each other, to care about each other, and if we argue or disagree within say a four- or five-hour meeting, that we don't take it out through the door and take it home, that we leave it within that building and that we don't leave as enemies; if anything, we leave more as brothers and sisters or friends as when we came into the meeting. . . .

There are water ceremonies which link us even closer to the environment of Mother Earth. Water is a purification liquid and we talk about it to our young people or to anyone that will listen; water is to be respected because it is life-giving like food. And to teach our young people how fortunate we are that we have water that we can still kneel down to, any stream almost, and still drink the water. Now, in some places I agree that it's not as good as it should be, but that's because of the kind of lives that we live and the things that we put on Mother Earth. The chemicals that we use in some instances growing the food that we eat is also destroying the things that we take for granted.

So those are the kind of spiritual healing things that we talk about and continue to help to grow and to understand a little better.

Case B: Mrs. Brown's Work-Related Allergy

Mrs. Brown visited her homeopathic practitioner, Dr. Gold, whom she had been seeing for some time about a skin allergy. Between Dr. Gold and a physician specialist in allergy, she felt her problem was under control. Now, however, she found herself, for the past two weeks, short of breath both at work and at home. As far as she could tell, nothing in her life had changed. Dr. Gold thought her condition sounded like asthma and he questioned Mrs. Brown very carefully. The only change in her life seemed to have been that Mrs. Brown was given a new job—processing snow crab—at the fish processing plant where she worked.

Subsequently, in conjunction with the allergy physician, it was determined that Mrs. Brown's problem was probably occupational asthma due to airborne snow crab antigen. It also became clear that the plant was taking insufficient precautions to prevent the antigen from becoming an occupational hazard. What should both practitioners do about the situation?

QUESTIONS AND COMMENTS

- What considerations must be taken into account when analyzing ethical dilemmas about our environment?
- What relationships do you see between aboriginal concepts of health and healing and complementary/alternative medicine?

- Is there a special relationship between environmental matters and complementary/alternative medicine?
- What response do you have to the groundswell of concerns about our environment?

Case A is a reminder that aboriginal ceremonies serve as ways of offering respect to people, the land, and the environment in general. Further, the ceremonies help to bring about healing. We have emphasized (see As a Healer in Chapter 7) the importance of connections in healing, and this is well exemplified in aboriginal ceremonies.

Interest in the environment and health is pervasive in the complementary/alternative medicine movement, though with less emphasis on connections. Emphasis is more on environmental hazards even aside from the discipline of "environmental medicine" that straddles the complementary/alternative and mainstream medical scenes. In fact, some would say that, in some senses, environmental issues have shifted out of mainstream medicine. This is in spite of a long tradition in Western medicine, extending back to ancient Greece, that connects the environment and health. Dampness, wind, and geographical location, as examples of determinants of health, were pushed aside, especially after the late nineteenth-century establishment of the germ theory of disease. That is not to say that issues regarding sewage, adulterated food, and industrial waste have been ignored by medicine, but these tended to be compartmentalized as public health issues and not so much a part of general medicine.

Studies on the relationships between the environment and health were not entirely absent during the 1900s, though much of the interest post-1960s emerged from concerns about pollution.[2] Rachel Carson's 1962 book *Silent Spring* is rightly seen as a catalyst for much of the concern over a host of "new" chemical contaminants or toxins in the air, land, and sea that affect humans directly or indirectly.[3] Such concerns provide a backdrop for the emergence of new, albeit still contentious, diagnoses such as "sick-building syndrome," "reactive airways dysfunction syndrome," and "multiple chemical sensitivity," for which sufferers commonly seek complementary/alternative care.

A variety of professional/ethical dilemmas can arise over environmental issues. Case B, for instance, suggests that the fish factory will need to modernize, which might lead to its closure, although it is a principal means of employment in the community. Here, once the facts have been determined to prove cause and effect (not always easy), much consideration needs to be given to such principles as doing no harm, and justice, with respect to individuals and the community.

It is important, too, to have a sense of environmental ethics to recognize one's own preconceptions. For example, are the latter in line with (1) a human-centered approach (moral standing given only to human beings such that nonhuman species and nature as a whole are a means for human ends), (2) a life-centered approach (in which moral considerations extend to nonhuman species), or (3) an even more inclusive approach that includes the moral worth of land, water, air, and ecosystems?[4] Such positions challenge practitioners and their professional organizations and societies to consider their responses to environmental issues. Should all societies cover these in codes of ethics? Is the following statement in the American Herbalists Guild code of ethics adequate and meaningful?

> All AHG members should acknowledge that individual health is not separate from environmental health and should counsel clients to embrace the "Earth-centered awareness."

This raises challenges about destruction of habitats of medicinal plants and their over-collecting.[5] To what extent should Plant Watch, which promotes sustainable harvesting of medicinal plants, be supported by complementary/alternative practitioners?

NOTES

1. From M. Joe, *Reflections on the Micmac Community of Conne River* (eds. R. Andersen and J. K. Crellin), St. John's, Faculty of Medicine, Memorial University of Newfoundland, 1996, pp. 16-17.

2. F. Sargent II, *Hippocratic Heritage: A History of Ideas About Weather and Human Health*, New York: Pergamon Press, 1982.

3. R. Carson, *Silent Spring*, Boston: Houghton Mifflin, 1962.

4. See "Environmental Ethics," in W. T. Reich, ed., *Encyclopedia of Bioethics*, New York: Simon and Schuster Macmillan, 1995, Volume 2: 676-694.

5. Compare M. J. Balick, "Transforming Ethnobotany for the New Millennium," *Annals Missouri Botanical Garden*, 1996; 8, 58-66; For other relevant comments: G. Lontz, "Coneflowers' [Echinacea] Popularity: Prescription for Trouble," *National Wildlife*, 1997; May 18, 12-13.; L. Thornton, "The Ethics of Wildcrafting," *The Herb Quarterly*, Fall 1998, pp. 41-46.

Testimonials and Advertising by Practitioners

ISSUES

- Testimonials: How should we approach them?
- Anecdotal information: What is its relevance?
- The impact of advertising

Case A is taken from an advertising section in a national magazine promoting naturopathic medicine, Case B is a patient's testimony circulated at public meetings on complementary/alternative medicine, and Case C is a practice advertisement.

Case A: Advertisement for Naturopathic Medicine

Max Zidel was three months old when he developed chronic ear infections. A series of medical specialists prescribed antibiotics for the Toronto boy. Then came the operations. By the age of five, Max's ear had been surgically drained eight times.

Finally, his mother, Denise, visited Thornhill, Ontario, ND Pat Rennie. "I hadn't lost faith in conventional medicine, but I was desperate," she explains. Rennie recommended that sugar, yeast, and dairy products be eliminated from Max's diet. She prescribed echinacea to boost his immune system and suggested massage to promote drainage and warm compresses to relieve pain.

The results were dramatic. "Max's infections cleared up almost immediately and he's had just one recurrence in the past 22 months," says Zidel.[1] (Reprinted from *Maclean's*, June 7, 1999, "You and Your Naturopathic Doctor" Advertising Supplement.)

Case B: "Cancer Can Be Reversed" by Angus Sullivan

It was July 1996—the beginning of a big change in my life. I had read an article in a health magazine on prostate cancer, stating that the routine check-up of every male over fifty years of age *should* include a P.S.A. (Prostate Specific Antigen) test. The P.S.A. is a marker or blood test for the detection of Prostate Cancer.

Being within the age bracket mentioned and due for my annual check-up, I requested that my doctor do a P.S.A. test, in addition to the usual D.R.E. (Digital Rectal Exam) which I routinely had had for the previous four years. Even though I was not experiencing any symptoms of prostate problems my doctor complied with my request.

My P.S.A. test showed a reading of 7.2 (normal is 0-4). I was referred to a urologist for further assessment, which resulted in a biopsy. The biopsy results showed that there was no cancer activity present in the prostate at that time. The urologist stated that another P.S.A. test would be necessary in six months. It was set for January 1997. This time my P.S.A. resulted in a reading of 9.2 which warranted another biopsy. In March 1997 a biopsy and ultrasound showed that I had localized prostate cancer with a Gleason core of 4.5 which indicated a mild to moderate malignancy. I was devastated with the news.

My urologist recommended immediate removal of the prostate and sent me home with video tapes and literature on "conventional" treatment. This treatment included prostatectomy, radiation, orchiectomy, hormone therapy, chemotherapy and watchful waiting. In addition to studying all this I spent the next several weeks engrossed in whatever literature I could find on prostate cancer. I tapped into resources at the Bliss Murphy Cancer Clinic, the National Cancer Research Society and on the Internet.

From my search I discovered statistics which showed that 50 percent of patients who have the cancer removed develop cancer again . . . *actually the Canadian Cancer Society's definition of "cure" is being cancer-free for five years only.* I was not impressed with these findings. Actually, I was terribly disappointed and felt that "conventional treatment" definitely wasn't the route I wanted to go. I kept searching for a better way and prayed that God would lead me to a decision I could "live" with.

My next few weeks were spent researching "alternative or complementary" medicine and its success rate in treating cancer. I discovered that the "alternative medicine" route uses safer, noninvasive ways of successfully treating cancer, using naturopathy, acupuncture and homeopathy. These were fields of medicine long recognized for their nontoxic holistic approach to treatment.

These methods were proven to destroy cancer cells *plus* treat the whole body and encourage the immune system to work at its full potential, achieving a level of wellness which helps to prevent or reverse cancer or any disease in the body. As a result of my research into alternative medicine I also learned that *success rates were best if these methods were used as a <u>first choice</u> of treatment rather than being preceded by harsh conventional methods such as chemotherapy and radiation, which almost destroys your immune system.* The more educated I became in alternative methods the more I felt that this was the treatment that felt right for me. I made my choice and took the path which today is frowned upon by most in the medical profession.

My first appointment for "alternative" treatment and therapy was with Dr. Gordon Higgins in April 1997; and as the saying goes, "since that time I haven't looked back." After the first month of treatment my cancer started to reverse, not by a lot *but* enough to give me hope. My appointments were scheduled 5-6 weeks apart and with the use of auricular acupuncture, Dr. Higgins would advise me of my progress and would treat other organs with homeopathic or herbal remedies as the need arose. His treatments addressed every facet of my life—mind, body, spirit, and emotions.

By December 1997, Dr. Higgins recommended that I see Barbara Sidel R.N., C.H.T.P. (Certified Healing Touch Practitioner) to help me resolve some childhood emotional scars which were preventing complete recovery. The healing touch therapy was successful in helping me. On January 29, 1998, Dr. Higgins informed me that *we had reached our goal of a cancer reading of zero. There was no evidence of cancer in my body.* Words cannot express how grateful Dr. Higgins, my wife Minnie and I felt at that moment.

Throughout my treatment period, at no time did I experience any discomfort or adverse side effects. I am experiencing a level of wellness that I have not experienced in many years. I am so grateful to God for setting me on the road to recovery. My advice to all who are diagnosed with cancer is to research "your" type of cancer; decide on a method of treatment that feels right for you; do all you can to help yourself and put your trust in God, and NEVER give up hope. While there is life, there is HOPE.[2]

[We have omitted the rest of the testimonial with specific advice on muscle relaxation, breathing exercises, and much more.]

Case C: Advertisement for Alternative Medicine Clinic

The following advertisement, typical of many appearing in local newspapers, was posted on notice boards in a mainstream health sciences center during 1998.

Acupuncture and Alternative Medicine Clinic
[name of practitioner] MD (China), D.T.C.M. C.S.T.
Specialist treatment for the following conditions:
Allergies
Constipation
Arthritis
Leukemia
Colon Cancer
Gynecological problems
Fatigue
Insomnia
Neck, Shoulder and Back Pain
Impotence
Spinal Cord Injury
Eczema, Psoriasis

QUESTIONS AND COMMENTS

- How important are testimonials in the promotion of complementary/alternative medicine?
- What arguments do skeptics of such testimonials use to dispute such claims?
- What professional/ethical issues are raised by practitioner advertising?

It is evident to anyone involved in complementary/alternative medicine that testimonials are an important way of encouraging interest in its various practices. At the same time, mainstream medicine readily dismisses them as anecdotal, giving them a very low level of credibility. To some extent this is colored by the long history of testimonials to support quack preparations with tales of faked and doctored testimonials.[3] Even the popular media recognizes the credibility issue from time to time: "Unorthodox healers rely almost exclusively on testimonials from satisfied patients. . . . Virtually every crystal healer and homeopath can cite people who report feeling better after their therapy."[4] Yet rather than dismissing testimonials out of hand, their pervasive role in all aspects of health care—they are also implicit or explicit in much advertising—needs to be fully recognized. To be totally dismissive of testimonials raises questions as to whether one is dismissing a patient's view of outcomes or, at least, sees them as overly optimistic. As Skloot said (see case history/reading 3), "sick people [seem] driven to reach out to a fellow sufferer." Because of the pervasive concerns over testimonials, practitioners have a particular responsibility to assess them critically if they use them to support a practice. The issue of raising false hopes in patients always exists.

Some of the concerns with testimonials apply equally to advertising. The tentacles of commercialism and entrepreneurship, long a feature of health care, were more evident in the late twentieth century as at any time in the past. Indeed, terms such as industrialization infiltrated health care, and tensions exist over whether health care and business are compatible. Moreover, there has been a change in attitudes among physicians from the time when they were prohibited from advertising—it was deemed unprofessional and undignified—except under a few specific circumstances; this avoided invidious comparisons between physicians and undue influence on the vulnerable sick. Nowadays, shaped partly in the United States by antitrust legislation,[5] views exist that "truthful advertising" not only serves to educate patients toward a more informed decision and choice regarding their medical care, but also, at least in the United States, enhances competitiveness among providers.[6] The essence of acceptable advertising is that it must be truthful and must be verifiable. Moreover, it should be the whole truth, in other words, there should be no omissions of material fact. Physicians must expect to be disciplined for violations.

Should complementary/alternative practitioners be held to the same standards? Is the advertising by many such practitioners, often along the lines of that in Case C, acceptable? Clearly, various professional/ethical issues arise, all the more so if the practitioner is unlicensed (as in Case C) and not accountable to any disciplinary process. Given the explicit references in the advertisement to conventional diagnoses (not traditional Chinese diagnoses), the advertisement may be interpreted as practicing medicine without a license. Although it only makes reference to treatment, many people may well assume the practitioner is competent to make the diagnoses listed. Further, the advertisement may raise false hopes merely because it identifies various conditions for which mainstream medicine has relatively little success.

An additional matter is the appearance of the advertisement on a health science center public notice board. Moreover, it was date stamped to indicate it had been seen by the administration. No disclaimer was attached to indicate that the institution took no responsibility for the information on the board. Could this be seen as validating the advertisement and encouraging the practice of medicine without a license? Might this influence a patient undergoing conventional treatment for one of the conditions listed? What responsibilities do institutions have?

Another issue—a general one rather than relevant to the specific advertisement—is the assessment of qualifications of the advertising practitioner. Without a register of practitioners, it is virtually impossible for any member of the public to check on the validity of a listed overseas qualification [e.g., MD (China)]. Moreover, other abbreviations are generally unknown or may be quite worthless.

We repeat that health matters highlight vulnerability and that professional/ethical issues rest on truth, the whole truth, and verifiability.

NOTES

1. "The Natural Alternative: You and Your Naturopathic Doctor," Reprinted from *Maclean's,* June 7, 1999, "You and Your Naturopathic Doctor" Advertising Supplement.

2. Circulated as a flyer in local health stores, and published in *Hope: The Alternative Magazine for Cancer Patients,* 1998; 2(2), 7-9. Reprinted by permission.

3. Compare J. H. Young, *The Toadstool Millionaires: A Social History of Patent Medicines in America Before Federal Regulation,* Princeton, NJ: Princeton University Press, 1961, pp. 188, 213-214.

4. "Faithful Flock to 'Cures,' but Scientists Want Proof," *The Toronto Star,* January 23, 2000 (available from the Internet site <http://king.thestar.com/the star/editorial/health/20000123NEWOld_CI-TRUST23.HTML> (accessed September 2001).

5. For outline of issues, W.T. Reich, ed., "Advertising," *Encyclopedia of Bioethics,* New York: Simon Schuster Macmillan, 1995, Volume 1, pp. 76-79.

6. "Statement on Ethical Advertising," Texas State Board of Medical Examiners Positions, available at Web site <http://www.tsbme.state.tx.us/guidelines/sea.htm> (accessed September 2001).

–8–

Making Diagnoses

ISSUES

- Who should make a diagnosis?
- Differences in diagnostic approaches between complementary/alternative and conventional practitioners.

We have already made clear the contentious issue of complementary/alternative practitioners making diagnoses. Here readers can explore relevant issues.

Case A: "Ex-Cancer" Patient's Stiff Neck

An acupuncturist, Dr. Peters (practicing in a jurisdiction that did not offer licensure) was visited by an "ex-cancer" patient, Mrs. Jones, who wanted treatment for a stiff neck. Dr. Peters, however, on the basis of "intuition" (clinical judgment) felt that something was not "quite right" with the way Mrs. Jones was holding her neck and asked her to get an X-ray before she could consider treatment. This was done privately by a chiropractor, who reported no abnormal findings. Unhappily, before the acupuncturist could reassess the situation, the patient was hospitalized in a coma. The acupuncturist heard that this was due to spread of the cancer.

The acupuncturist, in subsequently being "thankful" that she had not started treatment, wondered about the possible consequences, perhaps a malpractice suit.

Case B: Nonmainstream Testing and Diagnosis for Allergies

Mr. Sid Jones, forty-five years old, was feeling generally lethargic and often a little bloated. This condition had been present for about a year. If anything, it had worsened in the late spring. His life at home was "OK," but not very spirited. He had a checkup (with complete physical examination) with his family practitioner three months ago and no reason for his lethargy was found. Jokingly, his doctor suggested it was the male menopause, and that Mr. Jones should try to increase his exercise. Mr. Jones then heard from a colleague at work that there was a new alternative practitioner in the neighborhood (he was not sure whether he was a naturopath or not), who had helped a friend of his through change in diet.

Mr. Jones visited the alternative practitioner, who, after taking a detailed history, felt that they should consider a "food allergy," as a cause of lethargy and bloatedness. He confirmed this with two tests. The first was a muscle strength test (applied kinesiology) using a number of glass vials, each of which contained a food allergen. He placed each vial, in turn, on Mr. Jones' skin and identified the causative allergen as the one in the vial that "produced" the greatest weakening of the strength in an outstretched arm of Mr. Jones. The "weakness" was assessed by the level of difficulty in pressing Mr. Jones' outstretched arm down to his side.

In test 2, the practitioner used an electrodermal analysis with a Vegatest machine that measured the electrical resistance of a patient's skin. The patient holds one electrode which is connected to the Vega machine. A second electrode is applied to the patient's toe. The food allergen is placed in a glass vial on the machine, i.e., into the electrical circuit between the skin and a galvanometer. A change in skin electrical resistance is considered to indicate an allergic response to the allergen.

On the basis of the diagnosis, Mr. Jones was given a list of foods to avoid.

QUESTIONS AND COMMENTS

- Are lessons to be learned from Case A? Why is the thought of malpractice raised?
- What issues arise in making diagnoses through nonmainstream tests for allergy?

Case A

The concern regarding complementary/alternative practitioners making diagnoses has been raised in Chapter 4, under Safety and Standards. A particular issue in Case A (and we are aware of analogous ones) is, given that conventional medicine is mainstream health care in Western countries, does a complementary/alternative practitioner have a responsibility to ensure that a recent conventional diagnosis or an update on a serious condition is available? With hindsight, the acupuncturist believes that if she had started treatment, questions about her competency would have been raised. After relating the case to us, the practitioner said it was important to have some training in medicine (clinical and basic science, including anatomy), especially to appreciate how technology can offer help unavailable in complementary/alternative modalities (compare also Education, in Chapter 5).

Case B

"The allergy patient is increasingly caught in the tug-of-war between allopathic and 'alternative medicine,' pharmacists, so-called 'natural healers,' patient and consumer organizations, and the mass media."[1] In the context of such genuine concerns, along with the growth of general worries about environmental pollution, etc., physicians often fear that nonspecific ailments are often "misdiagnosed" as allergies or hypersensitivities by using such allergy tests as mentioned in Case B.[2] For instance, aside from the two tests mentioned there, another particularly contentious one that has become widely used in clinical ecology (a discipline generally viewed as alternative) is called "provocative neutralization" or "end-point titration." A test antigen is administered (sublingually or intracutaneously), a wheal response is measured, and symptoms noted (e.g., headache) that are viewed as an allergic response. Other doses are then given that "neutralize the original reaction." Potentially fatal responses have been noted.[3]

Integrated care is needed regarding allergies as reflected in the opening quote in the last paragraph. It is difficult to see any agreement being reached over nonmainstream tests without a full and thorough debate and clinical investigations on the differences between the diagnostic methods used by complementary/alternative and conventional practitioners.

Many other issues need to be addressed in connection with diagnosis, although they cannot be explored here. We mention only the seemingly greater readiness of complementary/alternative practitioners compared to conventional physicians to accept diagnostic labels for new conditions (e.g., hypoglycemia, chronic fatigue syndrome), conditions that many skeptics see as diseases of fashion.[4]

NOTES

1. B. Wuthrich, "Allergology: Quo Vadis?" *Schweizerische Medizinische Wochenschrift,* 1999; 129, 905-914.

2. See A. I. Terr, "Controversial and Unproven Methods in Allergy Diagnosis and Treatment," in R. Patterson, ed., *Allergic Diseases Diagnosis and Management,* Philadelphia: Lippincott, 1993, pp. 815-835.

3. D. L. Jewett, "A double-blind study of symptom provocation to determine food sensitivity," *New England Journal Medicine,* 1990; 323, 429-433. Concerns have continued.

4. It is of interest that the courts have been involved in the acceptance of the condition: K. Capen, "Chronic Fatigue Syndrome Gets Court's Nod of Approval As Legitimate Disorder," *Canadian Medical Association Journal,* 1998; 159, 533-534. See also H. Johnson, *Osler's Web: Inside the Labrynth of the Chronic Fatigue Syndrome Epidemic,* New York: Penguin Books, 1996, for insights into the acceptance of a diagnostic rather than clinical entity.

9

Prescribing and Selling Remedies

ISSUES

- Are there conflicts of interest?
- What is in the public's best interest?

Mrs. Smith visited an acupuncture clinic that she had attended fairly regularly for two years whenever she felt "wound up." She blamed this on menopause. This time her acupuncturist, Dr. Young, had added to his office a shelffull of Chinese herbs, mostly in capsules, and as single herb or combination remedies. Dr. Young told Mrs. Smith that she was advising some of her patients to take herbs along with acupuncture. The herbs, she added, were imported from China. Mrs. Smith wondered about ginkgo, since she thought she was becoming more forgetful, but also wondered whether it was cheaper to buy it at the drugstore. Dr. Young said that it probably was, but said that she could guarantee the quality of the products she stocked.

QUESTIONS AND COMMENTS

- Identify issues or potential issues in this scenario.
- What evidence might there be that imported herbs from China are good quality?

One issue in the scenario is whether a conflict of interest occurs in selling products from an office, a common practice. After all, although it was once common for rural physicians in English-speaking countries to dispense their own prescriptions, drugstores or pharmacies now shoulder the dispensing role. This, it is argued, provides a double check on the safety of the prescription, as well as allowing the patient a chance to ask another professional for more information. Concerns linger over physicians who have the power to prescribe, dispense medicines, and write death certificates (although this probably did not account for the separation of the first two activities). While signing death certificates is not a consideration for nonmedical complementary/alternative practitioners, dispensing from their offices means that one form of "checks and balances" in mainstream health care over quality and the power of practitioners does not clearly exist.

On the other hand, genuine concerns arise over quality of products as we have emphasized and Chinese herbs imported into the West have commonly been shown to present a health hazard. Complementary/alternative practitioners can argue justifiably that it is difficult to ensure that patients get consistent quality or even active products. As one chiropractor recognized in 1998, "pharmacists are very under-educated" and thus if a chiropractor felt strongly about directing a patient to a quality product "it isn't necessarily a bad idea" to sell it in his or her office and monitor the patient's response and progress. In response to the question, "What kind of ethical practice is that?" the chiropractor felt that until quality and educational issues had been resolved office sales were not a problem.[1] However, the worry remains that practitioners tend to look to larger profit margins than, say, pharmacists or, at least, chain drugstores. This can well be the case given the relatively small turnover of products in offices. Moreover, how do practitioners guarantee the quality of their products as did Dr. Young? This may not be easy, and her claim could be questioned; presumably she did not do her own quality control, and could only rely on the integrity of her suppliers.

Special Products

One reason for the office sale of products is to provide those not readily available elsewhere. Perhaps these are dried herbs, because a practitioner recommends only the whole plant rather than extracts that selectively isolate constituents. Some add that herbs are generally safe if they are used whole, or as whole extracts. A typical statement reads, "As soon as you start [selectively] extracting [a Chinese herb] and applying some of the information and the efficacy, you actually isolate the toxicity as well."[2] Representatives of ethnic groups and others often make the same general point when they focus on "a severe lack of understanding by mainstream physicians." As an aboriginal spokesperson said, "First Nations have used preparations of plant medicines and herb mixtures that, used alone, might be considered toxic, but used in the right combinations with other herbs and other plants, the plant properties negate the harmful effects and potentiate the benefits."[3]

NOTES

1. House of Commons Standing Committee on Health Minutes, April 2, 1998, p. 8.

2. Ibid., Feb. 10, p. 10.

3. Ibid., February 12, 1998, p. 7.

10

Critical Appraisal:
Toxicities and Clinical Trials

ISSUES

- Responsibilities in critical appraisal
- Responsibilities in counseling

Although we have stressed that determining the "facts" is a prerequisite in any professional/ethical decision-making process, this is often not straightforward. Just as medical students and physicians are now offered courses on critical appraisal, all practitioners must consider making this part of their lifelong learning. Critical appraisal has been highlighted in recent years through the advent of the Cochrane Collaboration, mentioned earlier, that has established protocols to be followed in appraising clinical research papers. In this case history/reading, while we do not have space to provide papers for review, we offer some comments on a paper which raises questions about decisions over conceptual matters.

Toxicities: "The Comfrey Controversy"

The debate over whether comfrey is safe has waged for many years and continues into the twenty-first century. Although it is easy to find testimonials, especially on the Internet, that indicate comfrey can be taken—in a salad, as a beverage, or as treatment for stomach ulcers, rheumatism, and other conditions—the medical literature points out the dangers of taking the herb internally because of the hepatotoxicity of the pyrrolizidine alkaloid constituents. External use as a compress for sprains and bruises is accepted, but even then only if the skin is unbroken. (The American Herbal Products Association states that preparations should carry the label: "For external use only. Do not apply to broken or abraded skin. Do not use when nursing."[1]) The debate is heightened by uncertainties, at least differences of opinion, about the amounts of pyrrolizidine alkaloids in the root and leaf (higher in the root) and differences between species and hybrids notably *Symphytum officinale* (comfrey), *S. asperum* (prickly comfrey), and *S. xuplandicum* (Russian comfrey) that appear on the market.

In the context of such issues, a 1996 academic paper, "The Comfrey Controversy"—which put forward the view that "scientific arguments against comfrey are inappropriate"—still carries currency.[2] The paper argues that there is a clash of paradigms:

> orthodoxy, on the one hand, demanding scientific proof of safety by the methods used for orthodox drugs; the herbalists, on the other hand, deeming current scientific methodology very crude and inadequate for measuring the fuller effects of the herb. If the role of the practitioner, individual response, patient enrollment—in short, all the trappings of the paradigm—are included, measurement becomes practically impossible.

Specific attention is given to the subjectivity of orthodox science, which is often overlooked, and that other "inadequacies" in scientific studies must be constantly kept in mind; for instance, such unsupportable assumptions tend to be overlooked as:

> the naturally occurring complex in the plant . . . can be regarded as a mere physical dilution of alkaloids and secondly, that the human metabolism is identical to that of the rat which is susceptible to these alkaloids, and not with the sheep which is resistant to them.

The author also notes that there are only four reported cases of toxic effects in humans and that the link to comfrey cannot be made without considerable qualification. She adds that "even where uncertainty is acknowledged, scientific opinion prevails," and gives as an example, the U.K. Committee on Toxicity report on comfrey:

> We recognize that the four case reports of human veno-occlusive disease are isolated and anecdotal and we cannot be completely certain of a causal link with comfrey ingestion. Nevertheless veno-occlusive disease is a rare condition and is often associated with the consumption of plants and seeds containing [pyrrolizidine alkaloids]. Thus we consider it probable that comfrey products were implicated in these cases.

In the conclusion to the paper the author states: "The science upon which the case against comfrey is based has not been carried out within the scientific frame of reference; it is not 'rigorous science' but lends itself rather to an interpretation as normative rhetoric." Readers need to review such papers carefully for the logic of the argument and how they can help with such questions as: Can I tell a patient it is safe to take comfrey?[3]

GENERAL COMMENTS

The comfrey saga underscores a number of issues raised elsewhere in this volume. For instance, the need to understand the different views about science, a herbalist's belief in the greater safety of the whole plant, and the use/misuse of the historical record. With respect to the latter, much of the argument that the danger of comfrey is overstated comes from the long history, the tradition of using the plant. In this case the "test of time" criteria (see Chapter 4, Critical Evaluation) needs careful evaluation, given the different commercial considerations of today and the way comfrey is used. Moreover, it is not clear that it has always been mainstream, at least among physicians. Although William Lewis' 1791 assertion that "many ridiculous histories of the consolidating virtues of this plant are related by authors" has been challenged at times, the negative views of physicians, expressed during the heyday of physician use of herbs, must always be examined critically.[4]

Given the uncertainties surrounding comfrey, offering advice to patients must mean giving all the information we have, making clear that uncertainty exists in the minds of many, and that alternatives to comfrey exist. We believe that information might well include animal studies, and the way ideologies shape interpretations. Although logic is evident in the comfrey paper, at issue, too, is the place of prudence in health care when definitive information is absent. Prudence may well be an appropriate approach to comfrey.

We have emphasized that clinical trials are a particularly important area for critical appraisal. Much advice is available on how to go about this, such as through protocols established for the Cochrane Collaboration. There are also specific professional/ethical issues that occur at various stages in a clinical trial, which should always be looked upon as experimentation on humans. Although ethical issues (e.g., informed consent, appropriate gender representativeness, inadequate attention to patient's concerns that develop during a trial) have been given increasing attention since the 1960s, they are far from new. We cannot resist a suggestion that Sinclair Lewis' book, *Arrowsmith* (1925, and the movie, 1931) be visited to follow the saga of physician Arrowsmith's failure to pursue an experimental treatment. He gave all members of a community a plague vaccine rather than dividing, as requested, the community into subjects and controls ("I did the humane thing; I lost sight of science.") Nowadays; much scrutiny exists in protecting controls in trials through the establishment of Ethics Review Boards.[5] However, concerns remain about the quality of trials undertaken by complementary/alternative practitioners, especially in office situations. For instance, are subjects given adequate information to give consent? Do they need to have the research and consent form submitted to an Ethics Review Board as do private physicians in many jurisdictions?

NOTES

1. M. McGuffin, C. Hobbs, R. Upton, and A. Goldberg, eds., *American Herbal Products Association's Botanical Safety Handbook*, Boca Raton, FL: CRC Press, 1997, pp. 111-112.

2. M. Whitelegg, "The Comfrey Controversy" in S. Cant and U. Sharma, eds., *Complementary and Alternative Medicines: Knowledge in Practice*, London: Free Association Books, 1996, pp. 66-84. Other quotes from this source.

3. Compare also C. Vincent and A. Furnham, "Complementary Medicine: State of the Evidence," *Journal of the Royal Society of Medicine*, 1999; 92, 170-177.

4. Quoted in J. K. Crellin and J. Philpott, *Herbal Medicine Past and Present, Volume II. A Reference Guide to Medicinal Plants*, Durham, NC: Duke University Press, 1990, p. 172.

5. It is important to recognize that concerns exist that stringency may limit what some researchers say are potentially important studies. In an influential 1963 paper A. B. Hill ("Medical Ethics and Controlled Trials," *British Medical Journal*, 1963; April 20, 1043-1049) said that in a controlled trial, as in all experimental work, there is no need in the search for precision to throw common sense out of the window. However, this view is debatable nowadays.

11

A Chronic Condition: Rheumatism

ISSUES

- Patients' beliefs
- Practitioner-patient relationships
- Rheumatology: Alternative treatments, quackery
- Case histories: What level of evidence do they provide?

One purpose of this case history/reading is to illustrate a chronic condition for which treatment shopping has become commonplace. By 2000, specialist rheumatologists had generally come to recognize that complementary/alternative medicine is a reality that must be "dealt with."[1]

Case A is drawn from a paper, which, typical of many published in mainline medical journals, is published as a "warning" about the dangers of alternative therapies. The location is Brazil, but the scenario could have happened anywhere. Case B is taken from another single case history of successful treatment of osteoarthritis with acupuncture. A key question for this reading is: How should one approach single cases, either published or presented orally?

Case A: Treatment Shopping for Rheumatism

The account is of a sixteen-year-old female who began to complain of arthritis, fever, malaise, and weight loss in October 1983 after a sports injury at school.[2] She was diagnosed as a case of polyarticular juvenile chronic rheumatoid arthritis (JRA) and started treatment with corticosteroids. Unfortunately, her condition worsened, and gold therapy and azathioprine were tried. She had a reasonable response, but for other reasons stopped this treatment. Her family "refused" surgery and decided to try "alternative medicine."

First, they visited a doctor well known in Brazil for practicing spiritualism. He prescribed spiritual sessions with no improvement. The family visited another practitioner who told them that he had special injections, prepared at his office, against *Brucella* which could cure the disease. This treatment commenced with intradermal injections of 0.1 ml. every three days. After twelve injections, the patient developed intermittent high fever (40°C), myalgias, nausea, profuse sweating, anorexia, and cough.

The authors next give a long list of laboratory test results after the patient was admitted to their hopsital; in the context of our interest here, this sharply underscores differences between "scientific" and "traditional" medicine. For instance, she was tested for a muscle enzyme (normal), agglutination for *Taxoplasma* (normal), mononucleosis (normal) and *Brucella*. The latter was positive at a titer of 1:160, two to four times higher than normal in the laboratory; a week later it rose to 1:320 (tube test for Brucella antigens Biolab-Merieux). In consequence, tetracycline and streptomycin were given and the patient had a good recovery.

In consequence, tetracycline and streptomycin were given and the patient had a good recovery.

In commenting on the case, the authors indicate that alternative medicine (including homeopathy) is commonplace in Brazil, and is a mirror of our "precarious" health system and the level of "general education in our population." They continue, "in this case, the family told us about the use of these intradermal injections only 5 days after the admission to the hospital," since they were afraid to acknowledge alternative medicine. The authors also note that the family refused to give them a sample of the injection for further studies.

Case B: Treatment of Osteoarthritis with Acupuncture

This case describes a fifty-six-year-old woman with a seven-year history of chronic upper neck and shoulder pain secondary to a diagnosis of osteoarthritis.[3] She had been having conventional therapy and a tranquilizer to control bouts of anxiety. She had been taking significant time off work because of pain and muscle weakness associated with her condition and her doctor had advised her that her next available option would be surgery.

However, on attending a pain clinic the initial treatment included maintenance on her normal medications, indomethacin (Indocin) 75 mg and alprazolam (Xanax) 0.5 mg, as well as acupuncture treatments and relaxation techniques. After approximately 6 weeks of this therapeutic approach, the patient's pain had diminished to the point where she was able to discontinue all prescription medications. Furthermore, she was able to return to work, resume all daily activities, and reported very little pain in the immediate follow-up. This patient has now been followed for an additional 5 years. She continues to come to our clinic two to three times each year for an occasional recurrence of mild to moderate pain, at which time she is treated with acupuncture as well as brief physical therapy. Most important, this patient has not needed surgery and continues to report a high degree of self-sufficiency in dealing with her condition.

QUESTIONS AND COMMENTS

- What contrasting issues are raised in Cases A and B?
- What is the value of single case histories?

Numerous surveys on rheumatic patients indicate up to 60 percent of rheumatology patients try complementary/alternative treatments.[4] All the reasons mentioned elsewhere to account for patient usage are relevant, but a particular issue is the inadequacies of conventional treatment including fears of side effects. In this context, the 1996 views of one rheumatologist remain valid in the early 2000s:

> It is perplexing that many physicians who care for patients with rheumatic disease vigorously develop and administer increasingly powerful and toxic drugs alone, and now even in combination, but dismiss without informed consideration the potential complementary role that safer, alternative forms of treatment might play.[5]

There is also optimism that some therapies—emerging from the castigation of complementary/alternative medicine as quackery—will prove to be clinically effective (e.g., use of glucosamine) for conventional use.[6]

Unfortunately, many practitioners (mainstream and complementary/alternative) find it difficult to decide on the best treatment recommendation for a particular patient, though there is always the tendency to favor one's own specialty. Just as Skloot was bombarded with suggestions for his Chronic Fatigue Syndrome (see case history/reading 3), many rheumatism sufferers find themselves in the same confusing position, a position compounded by intense commercial promotion. For instance, whether glucosamine hydrochloride is more effective dose by dose than glucosamine sulphate as claimed by at least one commercial producer.

Case A is typical of warnings, published fairly frequently in the medical press about alternative therapies. We suggest that certain physician attitudes may well be reflected in the report, as indicated by the following quotes: (1) "unfortunately, she developed side effects and stopped gold injections and steroid therapy;" (2) "the family told us about the use of the intradermal injections only 5 days after the admission to hospital," and (3) the family "refused to give us a sample." There is a strong possibility that the physicians failed to understand the family's beliefs and behavior, hardly conducive to quality care. It has often been reported that patients—at least in Western societies—are reluctant to tell their physicians about their use of alternative therapies. Unquestionably, special and sensitive efforts need to be made for patients to be comfortable in sharing such information.

The case seems to be one in which the complex medical scenario, indicative of the intimidating authority of Western scientific medicine, failed to offer a climate of trust. The physician authors rationalize the situation on the basis of, for example, poor economic and educational circumstances in Brazil, but this seems to sidestep the particular "refusal" by the family to have surgery or to hand over a sample of the injection. It is relevant to add that surveys of alternative medicine in Western societies, indicate that relatively high levels of education exist among users; any reluctance to pass on information to physicians suggests problems in practitioner-patient relationships.

What about the antibrucella injections? Is this mere quackery, which we define as deliberate fraud, rather than treatment which at least can be rationalized on the basis of anecdotal evidence and/or logic? Could it be seen as part of the long history of deliberately inducing fevers with organisms, in order to treat various chronic conditions (e.g., "General Paralysis of the Insane") or some variant of the belief that snake, bee and other venoms or stings can be useful? Could it be a form of cell therapy, though this is usually subcutaneous injection of freeze-dried cells derived from fetal tissues (commonly of rabbit or sheep). From the information in the paper one can only speculate.

Regarding Case B, as said, the popularity of complementary/alternative treatments for arthritis/rheumatism is linked to the limited success of conventional medicine and the side effects of its treatments. In fact by 2000, many see acupuncture as quickly becoming "mainstream," supported by consensus of its effectiveness in many areas of pain management.[7] Because of this, such single case histories can be seen less as anecdotal, but as further supporting evidence of efficacy. We agree with the authors' own comments on the case, that while "anecdotal" case studies are no substitute for controlled clinical trials, such information should not be completely disregarded when making clinical decisions.

NOTES

1. R. S. Panush, preface to "Complementary and Alternative Therapies for Rheumatic Diseases II," *Rheumatic Disease Clinics of North America,* 2000; 26(1), xv. It is noteworthy that this prefaced an entire 200 page issue, following another 200 or so pages on the same theme in the November 1999 issue.

2. From F. S. Cavalcanti and G. G. De Freitas, "Alternative Medicine in a Patient with Juvenile Chronic Arthritis," *The Journal of Rheumatology,* 1992; 19, 1827-1828.

3. From B. M. Berman and J. P. Swyers, "Establishing a Research Agenda for Investigating Alternative Medical Interventions for Chronic Pain," *Primary Care,* 1997; 24, 743-758.

4. For a recent review, A. Chandola, Y. Young, J. McAlister, and J. S. Axford, "Use of Complementary Therapies by Patients Attending Musculo-Skeletal Clinics," *Journal of the Royal Society of Medicine,* 1999; 92, 13-16.

5. A. M. Rosenberg, "Treatment of Juvenile Rheumatoid Arthritis: Approach to Patients Who Fail Standard Therapy," *Journal of Rheumatology,* 1996; 23, 1652-1656.

6. J. C. Delafuente, "Glucosamine in the Treatment of Osteoarthritis," in (Complementary and Alternative Therapies for Rheumatic Diseases II), *Rheumatic Disease Clinics of North America,* 2000; 26(1), 1-11.

7. *NIH Consensus Statement,* 1997; 15(5), 1-34. (Also "Acupuncture: NIH Consensus Development Panel on Acupuncture," *JAMA,* 1998; 280, 1518-1524.) The panel identified efficacy in postoperative and chemotherapy nausea and vomiting and in postoperative dental pain, and also stated: there are other situations such as addiction, stroke, rehabilitation, headache, menstrual cramps, tennis elbow, fibromyalgia, myofacial pain, osteoarthritis, low back pain, carpel tunnel syndrome, and asthma, in which acupuncture may be useful as an adjunct treatment or an acceptable alternative or be included in a comprehensive management plan.

12

Cancer

ISSUES

- Are there common features among all cancer patients who try complementary/alternative therapy?
- Special considerations for children.

Cancer and Adults

Case A: A Treatment Course for Breast Cancer

Monica Lewis, a forty-five-year-old lawyer, wife, and mother of three saw her family physician during September 1996. Upon self-examination she had felt something unusual in her left breast. She hoped it was a cyst but was particularly worried since she had lost her mother to breast cancer.

Upon manual examination, the physician also detected a lump, which he thought was suspicious in nature. A subsequent biopsy report revealed malignancy. Metastases were found in left axillary lymph nodes. Monica underwent a radical mastectomy of the left breast and axillary nodes. She was started on a regimen of chemotherapy.

On the suggestion of friends, she decided to attend the meetings of a support group for cancer patients. At the meetings Monica continuously heard positive testimonies of various alternative treatments which, as she witnessed, helped some of those present.

She asked her family physician's advice as to whether alternative treatments would be beneficial. He said he was very concerned about the use of alternative medicine by patients, largely because of false hope, but he admitted he knew very little about it. The physician recommended that Monica continue with the conventional chemotherapy and that he would help her check very carefully the evidence and safety of what was being tried. Monica did so, and, as she told her physician, she decided to try Essiac, which both agreed was safe. After finishing her chemotherapy treatments, Monica continued to drink Essiac tea, take mega doses of vitamins A and C, and to eat only organically grown vegetables.

In November 1997 Monica visited her family doctor because she was not feeling well. Investigations revealed that the cancer had metastasized to her liver. She refused any further conventional medicine. Monica knew the prognosis was poor and decided to try to maximize her quality of life as best she could. She decided to continue with alternative treatments, which would not involve hospital trips, IVs, or needles.

Monica used a regimen of coffee enemas and milk thistle. These were used to "clean out the filter of her body," the liver. It was suggested to her that if the liver were cleaned out properly, then it would function more efficiently, thus cleansing the rest of the body including cancer cells. During the terminal course of her illness, Monica's family physician made weekly visits to her home. Monica was usually in her bed. She was in a lot of discomfort and accepted morphine. Her husband took leave from work to help his wife. Each day the children, ages twenty-five, twenty-three, and twenty, would take turns spending the day or night at home with their parents to help.

During one of the doctor's visits to Monica's home, Kathleen, the eldest daughter, asked the doctor to pray with her mother and her. Recognizing how much comfort it would bring, he joined hands with the women and they prayed.

Two weeks later Monica died at home surrounded by her husband and three children.

Case B: Mainstream Medical and Homeopathic Treatment

A thirty-two-year-old woman, Sarah Brown, with abdominal discomfort, sometimes pain, saw her regular homeopathic doctor. Upon examination, Dr. Heinz palpated a mass on the right side of the upper abdomen. Suspecting a tumor, she recommended a complete physical examination by a physician, for she wished to have a conventional diagnosis before she would consider offering homeopathic treatment. Subsequently, a tumor in the liver was found and chemotherapy recommended. Before this was started, Ms. Brown called Dr. Heinz in a panic asking for advice. Dr. Heinz asked the patient to delay chemotherapy for two weeks while she started homeopathic treatment. This was done and by the time chemotherapy was started, pain, and tenderness were much improved.

Case C: Cancer and Children

Robert, a five-year-old boy in London, England, was found to have an extensive posterior fossa tumor distorting the floor of the fourth ventricle and extending downward into the cervicospinal cord to the level of C4/5.[1] The parents were informed that despite radiotherapy the prognosis was hopeless and that there was no further useful medical treatment. In searching for what to do next, they discovered a medical practitioner in the United States who felt he could possibly help or cure the condition. The treatment involved "antineoplastons" as anticancer agents, and the parents were provided with a list of publications in minor biochemical and oncological journals and a curriculum vitae of the researcher, detailing his considerable experience and expertise in the field of cancer research. In consequence, the parents decided to pursue the approach. As these drugs could only be administered through an indwelling intravenous catheter they requested that this be inserted in London for financial reasons. They also requested the supply of intravenous administration equipment.

The question for the physicians was whether they should collaborate. In fact they did so and inserted the catheter because, although there was no generally accepted scientific evidence that the treatment helped, there was no suspicion of toxic side effects or that the treatment did *not* work. Moreover, despite some risks in inserting the catheter, it was felt that it might help to improve terminal care, allowing Robert to spend more time at home if the treatment was unsuccessful.

The hospital also agreed to fund the costs of intravenous administration equipment for an initial period of three months at the end of which the child would be reviewed with a repeat MRI scan to assess the effect of treatment.

Unfortunately the treatment failed and Robert died.

QUESTIONS AND COMMENTS

- How common are the decisions made by Monica Lewis (Case A)?
- Should the homeopathic doctor have asked the patient to postpone the chemotherapy (Case B)?

- To what extent was communication between the two practitioners in Case B necessary for Sarah Brown's best interests?
- What are the special issues involved in cases of children with cancer and complementary/alternative medicine? Was it appropriate for the hospital to pay some of the costs?

No other interface between conventional and complementary/alternative medicine has aroused so much debate, as well as hope, as with cancer. A substantial literature has appeared that surveys the characteristics of patients who try nonmainstream types of treatments, as well as patient and practitioner attitudes. However, it is important to appreciate that studies have been undertaken in diverse places, from Australia to Norway, so that applying the findings to other geographical regions requires much caution.

Complementary/alternative practitioners can be involved in cancer care in various ways—from contributing to team care (perhaps as palliative care) to providing private care for a patient, who may or may not be using such conventional treatment as chemotherapy. Intense debate arises not solely because of poor prognoses, but also due to many cause célèbre "quack" treatments, some of which just "don't go away" (e.g., laetrile and the Hoxsey treatment), and new ones (e.g., from Italian physician Di Bella, 1998).[2] In this context, Quackwatch, the Internet crusade against quackery has extensive discussions on cancer with a "special message" to avoid the many alternative cancer treatments.[3] Cancer societies, too, raise many concerns.[4]

Of the various cancers, breast cancer has attracted particular attention in the 1990s, as part of the women's health movement. Complementary/alternative medicine has been very much part of this interest.[5] Many dilemmas have arisen for cancer sufferers because of the many choices; at least some of which—mind-body treatments, massage, touch therapy, and nutrition—have gained recognition as complementary care for cancer. In fact, these often have a key role where integration with mainstream care is evolving. As participants, complementary/alternative practitioners must recognize a responsibility to have more than their specialist treatment knowledge, but also counseling skills, an understanding of death and dying, the role of hope, and much more.

The story of Monica Lewis (Case A) mirrors many features that emerge from various studies, such as a good education, and a search for a quality of life while appreciating a poor prognosis.[6] Generally, most consult conventional medicine first (82 percent), while 15 percent start treatment simultaneously with alternative. Most patients, as did Monica Lewis, see complementary/alternative medicine as supplementary with hopes for improved physical resistance and improvement of their general condition. However, those who feel that they are given no hope or only very little hope of a cure from their physicians are more likely to use nonproven therapies.[7] She did tell her physician early of her interest and usage of alternative therapy, which perhaps fostered physician-patient relationships, and opened the door to discussion on potential safety and incompatibilities between various treatments. In contrast, reports indicate that many patients do not inform their doctors of their use of alternative therapies.[8] Calls exist for physicians to routinely ask questions, as part of history taking, concerning alternative treatments.

Monica's physician was not unsupportive, but, as is generally the case, did not open the door to what can be called integrated care. Nor did he really help with interpreting the confusing evidence about complementary/alternative medicine, though he did agree to pray with the family. As discussed earlier, spirituality is finding a place in mainstream medicine. If a physician feels unable to offer it, a responsibility exists to find alternative help.

Case B is obviously problematic for physicians, though homeopaths would not generally suggest postponing treatment. However, in this case Dr. Heinz was (1) concerned with the adverse effects Sarah Brown's present state of mind would have on her well-being, and (2) felt that treating symptoms early would be beneficial and that, once chemotherapy had started, the homeopathic treatment would be ineffective. She explained this to Sarah who agreed with the approach.

Case C is just one example of a number of heart-wrenching cases of minors (and their parents) opting for complementary/alternative medicine rather than conventional treatment. In some cases, the state, through the courts, has intervened, leading to state versus parents' rights confrontations. Media scrutiny has often led to cases acquiring international attention. One example is the Canadian boy Tyrrel Dueck, who died in July 1999; his case contrasts with Case B. In November 1998, he was diagnosed with osteosarcoma. Despite concerns on the part of the family, the parents agreed to a course of conventional chemotherapy. However, they and Tyrrel refused a further course in early 1999. The parents said they wanted to seek alternative therapy at a clinic in

Mexico. A subsequent court order resulting from successful application by Social Services mandated further conventional treatment. Unfortunately, before the order could be implemented, it was found that the cancer had spread and that further conventional treatment was considered futile. A stay at the Mexican clinic was fully covered by the media. After encouraging reports, Tyrrel returned home to die a short while afterward.

From information available through the media, it was one of confrontation, unlike Case B, in which, to a significant degree, there was a humane approach, a willingness to accommodate the hope of the parents. Although it cannot be said there was integration of care in the case, the physicians and the hospital were able to compromise in a constructive way. Although such negative outcomes are commonly interpreted by the media as failures of complementary/alternative care, the support they offer patients must be remembered, particularly in the context of studies that suggest "unproven" remedies make no contribution to five-year survival rates.[9]

NOTES

1. Adapted from C. Yeoh, E. Kiely, and H. Davies, "Unproven Treatment in Childhood Oncology—How Far Should Paediatricians Co-operate?" *Journal of Medical Ethics,* 1994; 20, 75-76.

2. The intense public and media interest prompted "official" medical evaluation, which concluded that there was no value to the treatment. Concerns have been expressed over the problem with the media of raising false hopes (R. Passalacque, F. Campione, C. Caminiti, S. Salvagni, A. Barilli, M. Bella, S. Barni, G. Barsanti, O. Caffo, P. Carlini, et al., "Patients' Opinions, Feelings, and Attitudes After a Campaign to Promote the DiBella Therapy," *Lancet,* 1999; 353, 1310-1314). Seemingly, too, a dramatic loss of public interest followed the negative results (U. Tirelli and F. DiFilippo, "Debate on DiBella Therapy," *Lancet* 1999; 354, 159).

3. <http://quackwatch.com> (accessed September 2001).

4. The Canadian Breast Cancer Research Initiative, for example, commissioned a series of reviews on Essiac, green tea, iscador, hydrazine sulfate, vitamins A, C, and E, and 714-X, and noticed weak evidence. Series begins with *Canadian Medical Association Journal,* 1998; 150, 897-902. Overall, the results called for more studies.

5. Many practices listed in H. J. Burstein, S. Gelber, E. Guadagnoli, and J. C. Weeks, "Use of Alternative Medicine by Women with Early Stage Breast Cancer," *New England Journal of Medicine,* 1999; 340, 1733-1739; R. E. Gray, M. Fitch P. R. Saunders, A. Wilkinson, C. P. Ross, E. Franssen, and K. Caverhill, "Complemen-

tary Health Practitioners' Attitudes, Practices and Knowledge Related to Women's Cancers," *Cancer Prevention and Control,* 1999; 3, 77-82.

6. For example, American Society of Clinical Oncology, "The Physician and Unorthodox Cancer Treatments," *Journal of Clinical Oncology,* 1997; 15, 401-406; A. H. MacLennan, D. H. Wilson, and A. W. Taylor, "Prevalence and Cost of Alternative Medicine in Australia," *Lancet,* 1996; 347, 569-573; S. D. Begbie, Z. L. Kerestes, and D. R. Bell, "Patterns of Alternative Medicine Use by Cancer Patients," *Medical Journal of Australia,* 1996, 165(10), 545-548.

7. For example, G. M. Shenfield, P. A. Atkin, and S. S. Kristofferson, "Alternative Medicine: an Expanding Health Industry," *Medical Journal of Australia,* 1997; 166(10), 516-517; S. D. Begbie, Z. L. Kerestes, and D. R. Bell, "Patterns of Alternative Medicine Use by Cancer Patients," *Medical Journal of Australia,* 1996, 165, 545-548.

8. T. Risberg, S. Kaasa, E. Wist, and H. Melsom, "Why Are Cancer Patients Using Non-Proven Complementary Therapies? A Cross-Sectional Multicentre Study in Norway," *European Journal of Cancer,* 1997; 33, 575-580.

9. T. Risberg, E. Lund, E. Wist, T. Wilsgaard, and S. Kaasa, "Cancer Patients Use of Non-Proven Therapy: A 5-year Follow-Up Study," *Journal of Clinical Oncology,* 1998; 16, 6-12.

Index

Abortion, 17
Abuse, sexual, 78, 115
Access to Medical Treatment Act, 24
Accountability
    in patient care, 30, 44, 71
    society and, 10, 112
Accreditation. *See* Education
Acupuncture
    Act (proposed), 97
    anatomical, 102
    asthma, 31
    case, 240-241, 243
    cost/benefits, 46
    education, 100
    opposition to, 8
    theory, 56, 75
    "unscientific," 21
Adams, Patch, 164
Adaptogen, 85
Advertising, 225
AIDS, 46
    organizations, 45
Allergy tests, 229
Alternative, 85
American College of Physicians, 24
American College of Radiology, 9
American College of Surgeons, 9
American Herbal Products Association, 235
American Herbalists Guild, 128, 154, 220
American Medical Association, 9, 117, 118
Anatomy of Dr. Nicolaes Tulp, 146-147
Antibiotic resistance, 183-184
Aromatherapy, 78
Arrowsmith, 238
Asthma, 31, 189
Atherosclerosis, 55
Attitudes. 55-56. *See also* Medicine, conventional; Professional
Authority. *See* Medicine, conventional

Autonomy
    individual rights, 20, 169
    patients', 19, 27, 95, 115, 150, 177, 215
    principle of, 131
Ayurveda, 55

Bacmeister, Theodore, 196
Balance/imbalance, 32, 33, 52, 53, 56
Battle Creek Sanitarium, 1
Baum, M., 57
Beecher, Henry, 129
Belgium, 96
Beliefs, popular. *See* Disease; Health care
Beneficence, principle of, 131-132
Biases, 7, 19, 50, 54, 55, 187
Bioethicists, tasks of, 5
Blaming patients, 169
Blood pressure measurement, 75
Blood-letting, 29
Bodybuilding, 194
Botanic medicine, 1
Brazil, 242
British Complementary Medical Association, 127-128, 183
British Medical Association, 9, 117
Brody, Howard, 115
Broyard, Anatole, 120, 146, 162
Business ethics, 45

Calcium-channel antagonists, 50
Canada Health Act, 63
Canadian
    Charter of Rights and Freedoms, 63
    health care system, 63
    Medical Association, 6, 117
Cancer, 22, 245-251
Candida, 53

Chaos theory, 56
Chaparral, 19
Chelation therapy, 192
Chemotherapy, 49
China, 59
Chinese traditional medicine, 52, 53, 56
Chiropractic, 9, 11, 99, 113
   economic benefits, 46
   opposition to, 100
   safety concerns, 77-78
Christian Science, 33
Chronic fatigue syndrome, 199, 230,
   242
Circumcision, female, 214
Clinical judgment, 116
Clinical trials, 29, 84, 237
   Cochrane collaboration, 31, 235,
      237
   meta-analysis, 30
Clinton, President, 43
College of Physicians and Surgeons
      of Alberta, 102, 115
   regulations, 24-26
College of Physicians and Surgeons
      of Manitoba, 26
College of Physicians and Surgeons
      of Ontario, 26, 45
Colonic hydrotherapy, 57
Comfrey, 19, 235-238
Common law in England and Scotland,
      104
Communication
   medical, 48, 97, 148-159
   nonverbal, 148
   teaching, 149
Competition, 8
Complementary and Alternative Health
      Freedom of Access Act
      (Minnesota), 104. *See also*
      Education; Informed consent
   children, 183, 189
   codes of ethics, 127-128
   competency, 100
   future, 10
   hospitals, 120
   licensing, 17, 20
   offices, 121
   professionalization, 113
   resons for use, 32-33

Complementary/alternative medicine
      (continued)
   research, 30
   science-based, 31
   terminology, 10
Confidentiality, 150
Consumerism, 4, 34, 104
Corporate power, 112
Costs. *See* Economics
Cuba, 59
"Cultural creatives," 53
Cunning Man, The, 21

Davies, Robertson, 7, 21
DHEA (dehydroepiandrosterone),
      191-194
Di Bella treatment, 248
Diagnosis
   by allied health workers, 118
   complementary/alternative
      medicine, 128, 132
   conventional medicine, 167, 225,
      227-230
   diagnostic classifications, 74-76
Dietary Supplement Health and
      Education Act, 19, 96
Dietary supplements, 19, 151. *See also*
      Herbs
   Canada, 3, 20, 47, 96
   cost, 45
   health claims, 96
   pharmacy, 28
   regulation, 95-97
   safety, 76
Digitalis
Digitalis lanata, 83
Digitalis purpurea, 82-83
Dilbert cartoon strip, 113
Discipline. *See* Medicine, conventional
Disease
   beliefs, 52-54, 242
   clinico-pathological approach, 119,
      148
   search for explanation, 203
Dossey, L., 161
Dueck, Tyrrel, 249-250

Economics, 41, 44-47
Education
    accreditation, 100
    basic science, 101
    complementary/alternative, 99-102
    continuing, 102
    professionalism/ethical, 2, 112
Efficacy/effectiveness, 85-86
Empathy, 158-159, 161
Empiricism, 52
Energy
    concept of, 52, 74
    energies, herbal, 84
Environment, 217-220
    ethics, 220
    medicine, 219
Ephedra, 19
Equanimity, 159
Ernst, Edzard, 10, 30
Errors, 73
Ethics
    "bottom-up," 134
    casuistry, 137-138
    consequentialism, 134
    feminine, 137
    feminist, 136-137
    of ignorance, 209
    principlism, 130-134, 186
    problems, approach to, 5, 111,
        177-178
    Review Boards, 238
    social utilitarianism, 134
    virtue, 135-136
    Working Group (U.S.), 43
European Commission, 34
European Union, 97
Euthanasia, 17
Evaluation, critical, 30, 33, 80-83,
    235-238

Faith healing, 33
Fédération des Professionels, Quebec,
    99
Feverfew, 84
Fibromyalgia, 47
Flat-earthists, 9
Food and Drug Administration, 3, 96
Foucault, Michel, 41

Foundation for Integrated Medicine
    (Britain), 60
Foxglove. *See* Digitalis
France, 96
Freedom of choice, 20, 32, 169

Gender, 136
General Medical Council, 6, 97, 112,
    151
    advice on duties, 123-124
Germany, 79
Gilligan, Carol, 137
Ginkgo biloba, 2

Hahnemann, Samuel, 117
Healing. *See also* Practitioner, as
        healer
    aboriginal, 219
    ceremonies, 217
    defining, 161-162
    medical schools, 161
Health care
    beliefs, 8, 32, 187
    concepts, 8
    shopping, 163, 167
    two-tier systems, 133
Health Maintenance Organizations, 167
Health reformers, 17, 28-29
Herbs/Herbal products, 28
    Chinese, 44, 232
    commercialism, 44, 83
    inferior quality, 76
    interactions, 60, 77
    lack of regulation, 83
    medicine, 54, 100, 117
        American aboriginal, 80
        diagnoses by herbalists, 75
        Traditional Chinese, 80
    prescription drug interactions, 77
    safety, 4, 19, 76, 80-83
    standardized, 84
    whole plant, 84
Hippocrates, 117
Hippocratic Oath, 116, 122, 124-125
History, 7, 18
Hmong refugees, 211

Holism, 4, 8, 21, 56-59
  practice/treatment, 1, 29, 33
Holistic science, 56
Holland, 9
Homeopathy, 48, 99, 117, 208-209
  case, 182
  computerized databases, 54
  economics, 46
  education, diverse, 100
  Homeopathic College of Canada, *xv*
  homeopathic medicines, safety,
    79-80
  licensure, 28
  otitis media, 185
  professionalization, 113
  theory, 29, 74
  "unscientific," 21
Hope, 57, 151
Hospitals, 119-120
House of Commons Standing
    Committee on Health,
    Canada, 28
Hoxsey treatment, 248
Humanities, 7, 48
Hypoglycemia, 230

Ideologies, 52, 101
  anti-establishment, 46
  conventional medicine, 9
  in science and medicine, 54-55
  two cultures, 8
Illich, Ivan, 41, 48
Informed consent, 23, 45
  complementary/alternative
    medicine, 154
  Human Rights Act, 152
Institute of Complementary Medicine
    (Britain), 79, 127
Integration, 2, 29, 31, 59-63, 101, 229
  in hospitals, 120
  models of, 61-63
  in prevention/public health, 168,
    169
Internet, 32, 33, 47
Interprofessional relationships,
    207-210. *See also* Team care
Iridology, 11, 76

Japan, 59
Jehovah's Witnesses, 43, 56
Jews and insulin, 56
Joe, Chief Misel, 217-219
Jonas, W. B., 60
Justice, principle of, 132-133

Keller, Konstantin, 79
Kellogg, John Harvey, 1
Kinesiology, 76
"Know thyself," 7, 146-147
Krop, Jozef, 22, 45

Lacombe, Michael, 114
Laetrile, 248
Listening, 149-150
Locke, Mahlon, 1, 58, 59
Lorenzo's Oil, 55
Lown, Bernard, 112

Malpractice, 71, 72-73
Massage, 28, 100
Matthews, Joan, 58, 98, 127
Medical Profession Amendment Act
    (Alberta), 24
Medicine, conventional
  art of, 116
  attitudes, 8-10
  authority and power, 9, 11, 114-122,
    242
  discipline, 6, 22, 105
  evidence-based, 30, 160, 195
  healing, 160
  institutions, 117-118
  oaths and codes, 122-127
  technology, 148
Metaphysics, 8,
Mind-body therapies, 78
"Modernists," 53
Multicultural health, 211-214
Multiculturalism Act (Canada), 63

Narratives, 177, 195
  as therapy, 204

National Center for Complementary and Alternative Medicine (U.S.), 3, 29, 31
National Health Service (Britain), 3, 61
Natural health products. *See* Dietary supplements
Naturopathy, 72, 99
Neo-Marxists, 41
Neurasthenia, 203
New Age, 56, 81
Nocebo effect, 87. *See also* Placebo effects
Nonmaleficence, principle of, 132
Nowlan, Alice, 196-199
Nursing, 27-28
    ethics of care, 102
Nutraceuticals. *See* Dietary supplements
Nutritional supplements. *See* Dietary supplements

Oaths and codes, 122-128
Office of Alternative Medicine (U.S.), 19
Ontario College of Physicians and Surgeons, 22
Osler, William, 121, 148, 159
Osteoarthritis, 239-243
Osteopathy, 48, 99
Otitis media, 181-186

Pappworth, Maurice, 129
Parkinson's disease, 22
Paternalism, 97, 131, 148
Patients. *See also* Practitioner-patient relationships
    patient-centered care, 22, 165
    rights, 23
    terminology, 11
Pellegrino, E. D., 135
Percival, Thomas, 125, 126
Pharmacy, 27-28
Physicians
    attitudes, 22-27
    responsibilities, 23
Phytotherapy, 84
Placebos effects, 20, 29, 86-88, 204
Plant Watch, 220

Plantain, 83
Platitudes, 149
Postmodern era, 5
Powell, judgment, 6
Practice standards, 71-73
Practicing medicine without a license, 74
Practitioner. *See also* Physicians; Professional
    as communicator, 148-159
    as gatekeeper, 167-168
    as healer, 160-163
    as health advocate, 168-170
    offices, 120-121
    as person, 146-147
    responsibility, 145, 168-169
    as scientist, 159-160
    as team leader, 165
    as team player, 163-167
    waiting rooms, 45
Practitioner-patient relationships, 154-159
    agency/engineering, 156
    collegial, 156
    contractual, 156
    fiduciary, 157
    friendship, 156-157
    paternalist (priestly), 155
Prayer, 11, 33
Prescribing from office, 231-233
Prescription drugs, 48
    interaction with herbs, 77
    side-effects, 48
Professional. *See also* Education; Ethics
    attitudes, 6, 8-10, 29
    being a, 5-7
    gender, 121-122
    knowledge, 116-117
    model, 11
    professionalism, 4
    professionalization, 28, 99, 113
    regulation, 97-99
    responsibilities, 1, 20, 44, 170
    roles, 6, 145-170
    traits, 113
    values, 6
Prognosis, 151
Pseudoscience, 17
Psychosocial care, 48, 57, 161

Quackery, 2, 9, 17
Quackwatch, 17, 59, 248
Qualifications, appropriate
    complementary/alternative, 226
    physicians, 102
Quality care, 7, 17, 55
Quebec, 99
Quinlan, Karen Ann, 129

Radionics, 76
Reductionism, 4, 8, 54, 84, 101
Reflexologists, 113
Reform, 34, 41, 43, 44, 45, 62
Regulated Health Professions Act
    (Ontario), 104
Regulation, 97-99
    ethics-led, 98, 128
    European Union, 97
    model, 96
    statutory, 98
Reibl v. Hughes, 153
Reilly, D., 87
Rembrandt, 146
Research, 30-31, 103
Rheumatism, 239-243
Rhinosinusitis, 22
Royal College of Physicians of
    London, 118
Royal touch, 1

Safety, 17, 47, 73-83. *See also*
    Standards
Saks, M., 8, 195, 204
Science
    fraudulent research, 159
    western, 21
Self-reflection, 7, 147
Silent Spring, 219
Skloot, Floyd, 7, 199-202, 241
Social contract, 112
Spain, 96
Spirituality, 8, 11, 33, 51, 163
    health, 161
    need for, 32
    New Age, 163
St. John's wort, 77

Standards, 83-85
Stone, Julie, 58, 98, 127
Switzerland, 96

Team care, 62
Telephone consultation, 210
Terminology, 10-11
Testimonials, 33, 48, 224-225
Texas State Board of Medical
    Examiners, 26-27
Thalidomide, 19
Therapy/Therapeutics. *See also* Holism
    drugless, 29
    healing/touch, 28, 223
    privilege, 151
    relationship, 98
Tierra, M., 76
Tobacco, 81
Toxins (autointoxication), 53
Traditional Chinese Medicine
    diagnosis in, 74, 225
    "language" of, 116
    theory, 52, 54
    tradition, 117
"Traditional Medicines," 96
"Traditionalists," 53
Truth-telling, 150
Tryptophan, 49
Two cultures, 34, 50-51

Unconventional Medicine Report, 34
Unionization, 99
University of Exeter Department of
    Complementary Medicine, 30

Values, 128, 135, 138
    in health care, 42-44, 46
    personal, 6, 187
Vietnam War, 19
Virtues, 145
Vitalism, 29, 52, 148
Vitamins, 96
    B$_6$, 51, 77
    supplements, 60
Vivisection, 159
Voodoo death, 88

Weil, Andrew, 22, 161
Wellness, 161, 168
Whistleblowing, 209-210
White coats, 121, 145

Women's health, 136
  movement, 75
World Health Organization, 56
Worldviews, 7

Order a copy of this book with this form or online at:
http://www.haworthpressinc.com/store/product.asp?sku=4536

PROFESSIONALISM AND ETHICS IN COMPLEMENTARY AND ALTERNATIVE MEDICINE

_____in hardbound at $49.95 (ISBN: 0-7890-1225-1)

_____in softbound at $29.95 (ISBN: 0-7890-1226-X)

COST OF BOOKS_____

OUTSIDE USA/CANADA/
MEXICO: ADD 20%____

POSTAGE & HANDLING_____
(US: $4.00 for first book & $1.50
for each additional book)
Outside US: $5.00 for first book
& $2.00 for each additional book)

SUBTOTAL_____

in Canada: add 7% GST____

STATE TAX____
(NY, OH & MIN residents, please
add appropriate local sales tax)

FINAL TOTAL____
(If paying in Canadian funds,
convert using the current
exchange rate, UNESCO
coupons welcome.)

❑ **BILL ME LATER:** ($5 service charge will be added)
(Bill-me option is good on US/Canada/Mexico orders only;
not good to jobbers, wholesalers, or subscription agencies.)

❑ Check here if billing address is different from
shipping address and attach purchase order and
billing address information.

Signature_____

❑ **PAYMENT ENCLOSED:** $_____

❑ **PLEASE CHARGE TO MY CREDIT CARD.**

❑ Visa ❑ MasterCard ❑ AmEx ❑ Discover
❑ Diner's Club ❑ Eurocard ❑ JCB

Account # _____

Exp. Date_____

Signature_____

Prices in US dollars and subject to change without notice.

NAME_____
INSTITUTION_____
ADDRESS_____
CITY_____
STATE/ZIP_____
COUNTRY_____ COUNTY (NY residents only)_____
TEL_____ FAX_____
E-MAIL_____

May we use your e-mail address for confirmations and other types of information? ❑ Yes ❑ No
We appreciate receiving your e-mail address and fax number. Haworth would like to e-mail or fax special
discount offers to you, as a preferred customer. **We will never share, rent, or exchange your e-mail address
or fax number.** We regard such actions as an invasion of your privacy.

Order From Your Local Bookstore or Directly From
The Haworth Press, Inc.
10 Alice Street, Binghamton, New York 13904-1580 • USA
TELEPHONE: 1-800-HAWORTH (1-800-429-6784) / Outside US/Canada: (607) 722-5857
FAX: 1-800-895-0582 / Outside US/Canada: (607) 722-6362
E-mail: getinfo@haworthpressinc.com
PLEASE PHOTOCOPY THIS FORM FOR YOUR PERSONAL USE.
www.HaworthPress.com

BOF02